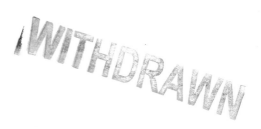

How to Build a Mind

MAPS OF THE MIND

STEVEN ROSE, GENERAL EDITOR

MAPS OF THE MIND

Steven Rose, General Editor

—

Pain: The Science of Suffering
Patrick Wall

The Making of Intelligence
Ken Richardson

How Brains Make Up Their Minds
Walter J. Freeman

Sexing the Brain
Lesley Rogers

Intoxicating Minds: How Drugs Work
Ciaran Regan

How to Build a Mind

TOWARD MACHINES WITH IMAGINATION

Igor Aleksander

Columbia University Press

New York

Columbia University Press
Publishers Since 1893
New York   Chichester, West Sussex

Copyright © 2001 Igor Aleksander

Library of Congress Cataloging-in-Publication Data
Aleksander, Igor.
    How to build a mind : toward machines with imagination / Igor Aleksander.
    p. cm. — (Maps of the mind)
    Includes bibliographical references and index.
    ISBN 0-231–12012–5 (cloth : alk. paper)
    1. Artificial intelligence.   2. Imagination.   I. Title.   II. Series.

Q335 .A44225 2001
006.3—dc21   2001017431

⊛

Casebound editions of Columbia University Press books are printed on permanent and
durable acid-free paper.

Printed in the United States of America

c 10 9 8 7 6 5 4 3 2

First published by Weidenfeld & Nicolson Ltd., London

Contents

Preface

> *Doth glance from heaven to earth, from earth to heaven;*
> *The lunatic, the lover and the poet*
> *Are of imagination all compact.*
> *One sees more devils than vast hell can hold—*
> *That is, the madman. The lover, all as frantic,*
> *Sees Helen's beauty in a brow of Egypt.*
> *The poet's eye, in a fine frenzy rolling,*
> *Doth glance from heaven to earth, from earth to heaven;*
> *And, as imagination bodies forth*
> *The forms of things unknown, the poet's pen*
> *Turns them to shapes and gives to airy nothing*
>
> *A local habitation and a name.*
> *Such tricks hath strong imagination,*
> *That if it would but apprehend some joy,*
> *It comprehends some bringer of that joy;*
> *Or, in the night, imagining some fear,*
> *How easy is a bush supposed a bear!*
> —William Shakespeare, *A Midsummer Night's Dream*

In my laboratory we are doing work that is called "reverse engineering" of the human visual system. My senior research assistant Barry Dunmall and I are puzzled by the way in which fifty or so brain modules, each made of millions of cells (neurons), give rise to very accurate visual sensations of the world. At the same time, the brain can imagine previously seen things or things that have never been seen at all. We are staring at his latest model which shows up on the screen of a computer. In terms of twinkling patterns, it shows the activity of every cell in a simulated (scaled-down) chunk of brain that includes visual and language areas. Barry sets the thing off and we can see its eye roaming around a simplified scene made of colored, stylized fruit, and some of the neurons giving a very accurate representation of the scene, while others are trying to describe it.

IGOR: So you have now separated out the imagination net from the perceptual one.

BARRY: Yes. Last week we were talking about how the model was going wrong because if you asked it to imagine things, its perceptual area was overwhelmed by the imagining and it was hallucinating rather than imagining.

IGOR: This then supports the idea that in the brain imagination and perception are physically separate. The evidence from brain-scans is a bit ambiguous. We must bring this up the next time we have our joint meeting with the neuroscientists.

BARRY: What's not clear to me now is how both these things come into consciousness. They are in different parts. We're losing a grip on what's conscious and what isn't.

IGOR: I think it's okay. If we stick to Francis Crick's idea that a neuron that contributes to consciousness must fire according to world-centered events, this still happens. The imagination neurons are producing imagined world spaces. So if I think of my cat while I am looking at you, the vision of the cat has a place in my imagined field of view, but because of the separation it does not "feel" as if you and the cat get confused—it simply feels as if the two are somehow simply happening at the same time. The model's coming good now, let's stick with it and start looking at positional imagination clues like "think of an apple to the left of the banana."

I only recall this recent conversation because it shows that words like *consciousness* and *imagination* have crept into the world of computational machinery in much the same way as *knowledge, memory,* and *intelligence* have done in the past. I know that some will approve and others will be horrified at what engineers are doing by using words in this way. In fact, I believe that, while much care needs to be taken when coupling words such as "imagining" with machines, disapproval should not prejudice the exciting insights into mental phenomena that prompted me to write this book. Not everyone can join Barry and myself in our laboratory, but, through this book, I describe how, over many years, we have got to a point where working with imagining machines is beginning to tell us how real imagination and consciousness might come about.

The joy of being conscious, for me, lies in the amazing sense of freedom that I feel is available to my imagination. My consciousness not only puts at my disposal an accurate perceptual knowledge of the real world, but also enables me to imagine what I want to do in this world and allows me to make up worlds and actions that I may never have experienced. While most agree that the brain is responsible for our sensations, most will also say that it is now known how perceptual knowledge gives rise to imagination. My kind of engineering contains some simple, easily understood principles that are there solely for the purpose of explaining similar cause-and-effect circumstances in machines. To keep things simple, and to avoid the "oily rag" image that the word *engineering* evokes, I have described in this book both a biography of my own understanding, and some imagined encounters with philosophers who created the backbone for what needs to be understood.

The trouble with philosophical discussion is that in itself it has become very technical. It is often burdened by many "-isms." *Dualism, reductionism, epiphenomenalism,* and the like have become the currency that circulates through some texts and burdens the airwaves during public debates. My consciousness is a joy for me and not an "-ism." When I approach our machines in the laboratory, that's what I want to know: how does the mechanism of my brain translate into the joy of my free imagination. The machine is just a tool that may help me in my quest. "Outrageous reductionism, scientific arrogance," someone once said to me. "You are ignorant of two and a half millennia of philosophy, you are flying in the face of what people wiser than you have concluded about consciousness."

I agree that it is very important to know what philosophers have said over this period of time. In my working life I took to reading about philosophy in parallel with the development of my engineering work, and I wish to reflect on this through this book. I believe that the likes of Thales of Miletus, Aristotle, Descartes, John Locke, Ludwig Wittgenstein, and many modern thinkers are driven by the same questions as I am. The difference is that we all have different tools and methods with which to produce some answers. I wish these thinkers to feature in this book not as austere intellectual figures, but rather as people who are using their own experience and the knowledge of their time to reflect on the nature of our mental lives. But how can my engineering experience with the machines of my time contribute to this? My late colleague Eric Laithwaite was very clear about this.[1] Many successes that engineers are proud of are present all around us as the products of natural evolution. Camouflage, the flight of insects, the vision of the night owl, are all more efficient than human technology at its highest. But the reason that even inadequate engineering is important is that it allows us to recognize and understand the working of complex machinery in nature and to use it as an inspiration for building useful machines.

And so it is with consciousness. This is a phenomenon possessed by living organisms which surpasses by far anything we can engineer in our laboratories. This is likely to be true for a long time, if not forever. But the process of developing progressively more competent neural machines has helped me personally to feel comfortable with how my brain might be causing my sensations. That which makes my consciousness different from that which can be built is an important part of the discussion. This difference holds some of the features of an explanation.

In addition to being an explanatory device, it is worth asking how such machine consciousness might also empower useful machines. The relationship between the artificial and real versions of consciousness remains just like that between the robot with vision and the night owl. The robot may be quite different, but understanding the properties shared by the two is sufficient to design robot vision systems inspired by the excellence of owl vision, and to understand owl vision better by knowing how robot vision can be designed. Not many would say that this diminishes our respect for the owl. So I hope that reading about artificial imagining machines built using human skill will encourage the reader to share in some of the excitement that Barry and I enjoy in playing with such machines.

Thanks

The fact that I have been able to write this book at all makes me grateful to more people than can be mentioned by name. At the time of writing I can list over sixty Ph.D. students without whom my own thoughts could not have developed at all. I also delight in getting the best family advice possible from a psychologist, a social anthropologist, and a biologist in the shape of Helen, Joe, and Sam. Their advice is not always on academic matters, but their fond tolerance for me and my bookish tendencies has been a joy for over a couple of decades.

How to Build a Mind

Imagination and Consciousness

Lights are Intelligences in our minds, whose force
We no more comprehend than here, in these
Glittering jewels, we can say how rose
Or sapphire blue or emerald steady shines,
Or what makes all the brilliant colours glow
Along the throat of the Arabian bird,
Whilst here, in milder air, her neck is grey
Or in the Polar void a brilliant white.
   —A. S. Byatt, *Possession—Mummy Possest*

I imagine therefore . . .

As I sit tapping the keys on my laptop, I notice the oval table on which
it is propped up with a newspaper so as not to wobble. The table is
"rustic." It's the kind that costs too much in an antique shop, but finds
its way to junk shops without too much difficulty. I look up and,
through a large window, I see the Mont Scholastique—one of the
many smoothly shaped tall hills of this part of the Languedoc. Pleasant memories of picnics at the ruined chapel at the top of the hill
flood back. I look through a smaller window to my right and see the
village of Octon across the cultivated valley of the Salagou River. Later
today Helen and I will swim in the Salagou Lake . . .

Believe it or not, there is some purpose in this reverie. The reminiscence is made possible by an astonishing mixture of things: perception, memory of occurrences and feelings, plans and expectations. I am imagining things and through the use of words hoping that anyone who reads this can, using their imagination, share with me some of these experiences or, at least, believe them to be possible. But there's more: we are all capable of fantasy and of appreciating the fantasy of others. Great literature, poetry, science fiction, the movies, the stage are all part of what makes our mental world not just a dry topic called "mind" but a matter of supreme importance in our existence. Mind is the place in which we live. We can imagine the consequences of the actions of despots, appreciate the acts of benefactors, and live our lives according to principles. We live by our imagination, we continually add to our imagination, we trade our imaginings. We *are* imagining organisms. But are we just specific examples of imagining machines of which there are many? Do animals imagine? Could imagining machines be made? Can we understand what mechanisms in the brain bring this imagination about?

The usual word used to describe our active mental experience is *consciousness*. As words go, I feel that this one is a little tired. It appears in acrimonious debates in philosophy and science. It appears in the titles of many books, it is shunned by rigorous scientists and abused by not so rigorous ones. It has one significance for the anesthetist (will the patient jump off the table when stabbed with a lancet?) and a completely different and differing set of meanings for philosophers. Unashamedly, I want this book to be about consciousness, its wonders and pleasures. But I want to avoid the yawns and the pointless late-night conversations about its elusiveness. For this reason, I look for the force of consciousness in the power of imagination. I need to understand how my brain, an evolved machine of awesome complexity, can provide me with not only pleasurable reverie but also all the other elements of my mental life.

Imagination: Engineering and Philosophy?

Admitting that I am an engineer is (in the United Kingdom at any rate) a bit like standing up at a meeting of Alcoholics Anonymous and confessing to the error of one's ways. The trouble with the word is that it is associated with oily engines. In some parts of the world it is associated with the word *genius*—but I am far too humble to stress this. Nevertheless, being an engineer has been enormously helpful to me in understanding some of the principles that must be at work in the brain. In this book I want to pass these thoughts on without requiring anyone to know about engines of any kind, oily or otherwise. The point is that working with informational machines (some, but by no means all, of which are called computers) I find myself designing machines capable of handling the kind of stuff that makes up our imagination.

"Can a machine imagine?" is therefore a key question. If it can (and, clearly, I believe it can), how does its makeup distinguish it from one that cannot? The answer will not be revealed in the next paragraph or two but, hopefully, will begin to emerge by the end of the book. I hope that the reader will then join me in what is no more than a glimmer of an understanding. A glimmer may not be much to promise, but for me it has been a great step forward from understanding nothing. It is for this reason that the book needs to be read as a bit of a journey: a journey through my own past experience, and a journey through what some others have said about consciousness. The story will not be one of sifting systematically through scientific theory, as would be the case with a learned text, but a tale of pennies dropping in some kind of chronological order and in the context of my own developing comprehension. The backdrop does not stop with engineering, psychology, and neurobiology. A crucial context for such an understanding is philosophy. Philosophy is not something I learned through an engineering education but something I picked up as a fascinated external observer. This too, therefore, provides resting stops in the proposed journey.

Machines I Have Known

Of course, I am not the first to have thought that an understanding of engineering can throw light on living organisms and their mental life. Many with similar aims inhabit the history of the twentieth century. In the early 1940s, the Massachusetts Institute of Technology (MIT) mathematician Norbert Wiener observed with some effect that the laws of control and information engineering which are used to analyze the automatic control of airplanes, rockets, and industrial plants apply to living beings as well. This became known as cybernetics and had a major influence in engineering, psychology, and management sciences in the 1960s. Also in the 1940s, the physician Warren McCulloch and the logician Walter Pitts, again at MIT, started making electronic models of brain cells and wondering at what point anything one could call "thought" begins to show up in networks of these. In the 1950s, British engineers Colin Cherry and Donald Broadbent became puzzled by the ability of human beings to attend to some things and filter out others. They modeled the processes using the electronic circuits of the day, and their models of attention have become central to the work of cognitive psychologists up to the present day. But these were clearly just beginnings. In chapter 3, I describe grappling with these ideas and trying to work out how much more needed to be done—it was a lot.

After a spell in industry and the completion of a Ph.D., I became a lecturer at Queen Mary College in London. I started to play with the design of single neurons. McCulloch had expressed himself in terms of the electronics of radio: volume controls, amplifiers, and the like. It would be inconceivable to build anything of any size in this way. Something had to be done in what was rapidly becoming a digital microcircuit age. But this was also the time that saw the beginning of the fashion for Artificial Intelligence (AI). Within this environment, thoughts of engineering inspired by the brain did not find a sympathetic hearing. In chapter 5, I describe how the computing world was becoming engrossed in making systems that seemed to do intelligent things, but where the intelligence came from the brilliance of programmers and the power of machines. I thought that this told us very little about how our own intelligence comes about. This was not a popular view. But I found the contrast between programmed AI and the ability of the neural networks in our brains—neural nets which might be investigated using the newest silicon techniques—surprisingly revealing.

In the late 1960s I moved to the University of Kent, which was then one of the "new universities." In the spirit of doing new things in a new university, I began making machines of a "neural" kind using the earliest digital microchips. The timing was bad as this approach was being thoroughly trashed by the Artificial Intelligentsia at MIT. Marvin Minsky and Seymour Papert published an influential book that elegantly destroyed the ideas of McCulloch and others about learning in neural systems, in favor of programmed intelligence. In chapter 7, I describe how this led to a trip to MIT, where rather than being convinced that the AI way was the royal road, I became even more deeply entrenched in my view that this approach will never satisfy anybody's curiosity about the brain.

However, another important penny dropped at that time: in order to have imagination, a machine must have neurons that interact with each other in such a way as to sustain their own internal encoding of things or embryonic "thoughts." In other words, they must have inner states (that is, firing patterns of neurons) capable of rich representations. An encounter with Stuart Kauffman, then a graduate student at MIT and now a recognized expert on emergent order in chaotic systems, led to the idea of these interacting nets of neurons having interesting emergent properties of their own. They have a neat way of arriving at their significant inner states in very few steps. This is pleasing because it correlates with most of our experience. Also, the contrary experience of, say, not being able to put a name to a face, has an explanation as a property that emerges under some conditions in a neural net. These are properties that feature strongly in imagining nonliving nets, and possibly their living counterparts. In fact, these internal state structures and their emergent properties are the first major features that distinguish machines that can imagine from those that cannot. Easily said—but understanding and controlling these properties became not only a difficult research task, but one that required a great deal of concentration and led to turbulent times in my personal life at Kent.

A further move in 1974 took me to a chair at Brunel University. Both pressure from funding agencies and the desire to do something useful led to the design of WISARD, an early neural pattern-recognition machine. In chapter 9 we shall see how this machine, using neural networks, could recognize patterns as complex as faces but, alas, had no imagination at all. This allowed another important principle to fall into place. People talk far too glibly about "recognizing" things and then build machines that simply label patterns. There is a vast difference between recognizing patterns by labeling them correctly and knowing the objects that are perceived. Such knowledge is a happy resonance between imagination and perception, possessed neither by WISARD nor by the many neural pattern-recognition machines built over the last fifteen or so years. Something extra is required: yes, inner states are necessary, but they cannot be just any old inner states.

Working with neural systems received a boost in the 1980s. It became fashionable in the United States again with the work of innovators such as John Hopfield at the California Institute of Technology who, in 1982, published an elegant theory of inner states in nets based on principles of energy. So my desire to do something about machines with inner states capable of imagination returned just as I made another move: to Imperial College in London. In chapter 11, I shall outline how MAGNUS, a machine driven by inner states, was conceived, how it has developed to the present day, and how it excited journalists. A spell at the California Institute of Technology with a group specializing in visual awareness in primates clinched for me those principles that are essential for a system to be able to become aware of its world and to be able to imagine it.

Philosophical Imaginings

My own exploration of machinery with internal states capable of imagination is one strand of this book. The other, as trailed earlier, is that I am encroaching on territory conventionally trodden by philosophers. I therefore felt the need to understand why my ideas might be running against conventional culture. Why do some feel uneasy about my mechanistic approach? Understanding the passions and opinions that are stimulated by the idea of artificial minds is almost as important as designing such artificial systems in the first place. Such passions are often quite explicit. I am labeled as a reductionist. I am often told that I am flouting philosophical areas of agreement. These views come from deeply held beliefs that have their roots in many millennia not only of philosophy but also of cultural evolution. It is vital that I should not ignore this existing wisdom.

But I am a visitor in the land of philosophy, and a visitor I need to stay. I would not dare to attempt a critical essay. So I have imagined being able to talk to, or just to hear, the influential philosophers of Western civilization on topics that relate to mind and its origins. In chapter 2, I imagine being a castaway in 540 B.C. in the region of Miletus where, by many accounts, philosophy began. The concern of Thales, Anaximenes, and Anaximander for answering deep questions about "what are things made of" does not stop at material things. The notion of a soul emerges. Does it survive the body? It is destined that our human sense of the enduring self will be central to the discourses of those who follow in the footsteps of the Miletians for thousands of years to come. The Miletians spoke of machines, but autonomous motion was for them what defined life. How valid was this as an idea at the time?

For me, the great era of Greek philosophy reached a peak with Aristotle. Here was a giant not only in the history of philosophy but also in the history of humankind. Through Saint Thomas Aquinas and Saint Augustine, he influenced the Christian culture that molds much of the way in which mind and soul feature in Western thought. But what might Aristotle have been like at the decline of his influence in his own time? In chapter 4, I imagine being a fly on the wall during Aristotle's trial for impiety which led to his flight from Athens. This fictional segment of the book lets me imagine how Aristotle may have viewed his own accomplishments, from the tutelage of Alexander the Great to his thoughts on the soul and minds of mortals.

Undoubtedly, another hugely influential figure in the history of philosophy was René Descartes, who is now more often criticized than followed for his division of mind from body. But, purely personally, I have been fascinated by the immediate effect that Descartes had on the philosophers who followed him after the end of the seventeenth century. Known as the empiricists, John Locke, David Hume, and Immanuel Kant were concerned not so much with how minds work but with what kind of objects they contain. How does an imagined idea differ from an experienced one? To imagine their reactions to the idea of an imagining machine, chapter 6 is a dream about these thinkers being subjected to the brashness of a television interview: an experience which many modern thinkers are forced to experience.

Hopping from giant to giant, in chapter 8 we meet Ludwig Wittgenstein on a train to Cambridge. I find him enigmatic but enormously stimulating. He was aware of the debate that was beginning to surround Alan Turing's idea that computers might be able to think. During the train journey I imagine that he has the opportunity of telling me how misguided I am for looking for the mechanisms of imagination in anything but the world of human beings.

The "expose it in the media" theme, started in chapter 6, is revived in chapter 10. "Consciousness" is the basis of many popular programs on TV and a vast number of popular books, and a source of robust public debate. I imagine being part of a millennial radio discussion program chaired by British media personality Melvyn Bragg. I am caught in the crossfire between scientists, philosophers, and mathematicians, all of whom have seen fit to pronounce on the nature of consciousness during the last decade of the twentieth century. What chance do I as a machine-builder stand in this array of eloquent dissonance? Does the imagining machine become the common anathema for the others? At least, I get a word in edgewise on how working with machines might throw light on opposing opinions.

So How Does Imagination Work? Is the Question Clear?

It would not only be thoroughly unprofessional for me to give away at this stage what I think to be the answer, but the answer itself would not make much sense without taking the journey that I describe in this book. It took me that length of time to begin to see some of the "Lights" that are the "Intelligences in our minds" so imaginatively expressed in Antonia Byatt's poetry. So I leave it until chapter 12 to approach the flimsy beginnings of an answer, while here I wish to focus a little on the exact nature of the question that needs to be answered. In doing this I recognize that whatever it is, it begs most of the questions posed by the puzzle of consciousness. I cannot avoid the word in my vocabulary, but I need to treat it carefully: it is capable of leading us back into culs-de-sac that have emerged over more than two thousand years.

To illustrate what might constitute an appropriate question, imagine that one day a robot arrives in town and everyone agrees that it is a conscious machine. We purposefully but temporarily put aside the question of how anybody knows that it is conscious. The designer of the machine proposes to tell us how its consciousness works. In what sense are we better off? This clearly depends crucially on how the designer expresses herself. Should the explanation be couched in a series of quantum-theoretical equations, we would have a situation where the quantum physicist says to the rest of the world, "I know how consciousness works but no one else can, unless they learn quantum physics." Similarly, a computational explanation might mean something only to the computer scientist, and a neural one only to the neural network expert.

Clearly, it is important that the explanation should make sense to common experience in the way that most of us can grasp what happens when water freezes, when a light bulb lights up, when a baby is born, or when the earth goes around the sun. So what is it that puzzles all of us about those inner feelings we call our imagination, our consciousness? I suggest there is one key question that dictates the underlying agenda for this book:

> What is there in my brain that allows me to feel that I, as an individual, live in a real world, can imagine without perception, know who I am, and am able to decide what I want to do?

This is the question that has motivated my work for a long time and now motivates the writing of this book

It Can't Be Done!

Some readers may have read this far with a mounting degree of incredulity. Have I not heard that American philosopher John Searle has said that computers, because they are programmed to use symbols, can never have the imagination necessary to understand natural language?[1] Imagining my rustic table is just what they cannot do: they can only manipulate "rustic" and "table" as meaningless symbols. Have I not heard that another American philosopher, David Chalmers, has shown that modeling the neural structure of the brain (as I do) can only get to grips with some easy side of the problem, leaving the hard part (the stuff of feelings and imagination) untouched?[2] Have I not heard that the brilliant British mathematician Roger Penrose has argued that consciousness is noncomputable?[3] Indeed, he has written that the answer lies in some form of quantum processing in the microtubules of the brain. Microtubules are those parts of the structure (cytoskeleton) of the brain that keep the neural networks of the brain in place.

It Might Be Done!

I have no quarrel with Searle, Chalmers, or Penrose. But I do warn the reader against believing that anyone, including myself, who presents their ideas on how consciousness works, has the last, definite word. The arguments used by Penrose are elegantly illustrated by showing that consciousness involves "insight." An example he quotes is the insight needed to decide how to prove a mathematical theorem. He rightly worries about the limitations of computation as we know it from our laptops. The point I shall make is that machines are not all like my laptop, and that some might well perform computations in other ways—ways that include insight, consciousness, and imagination. I argue for the existence of such machines while Penrose recognizes the limitations of current computational powers. Both are beliefs, but they are not contradictory and neither is the last word.

David Chalmers, on the other hand, may be importing an error from the philosophical deliberations of several millennia. For this reason, some of the great Greek philosophers appear in this book: they had few scientific facts at their disposal, and some believed that the philosophy of the mind should be based on the power of the mind turned on itself rather than its physical character. Anticipating subsequent discussions a little, the "hard problem" is this: It may well be that, put in a suitable magnetic resonance imaging (MRI) apparatus (a brain-scanner), the thoughts of a subject could be found to correlate exactly with the broad activity of the brain that the experimenter can see on the screen. The "easy problem" is to construct theories of how such brain activity is generated, learned, and modified. The "hard problem" is to work out how this activity *causes* anything the subject might *feel* internally. Some philosophers object to those who say that the two are the same thing, and call them "reductionists." The latter retaliate by calling the former "dualists" (there are many "-ists" in between, which need not concern us for the time being). However, as the relation of brain activity to sensation is becoming progressively better understood, it seems to be a tiny bit perverse to relegate for eternity such findings to some "easy" category, believing that the "hard" unyieldingly shifts further afield.

For most, such distinctions are pretty distant. But on the whole, the instinct of many would lean toward dualism rather than reductionism, for purely cultural or historical reasons. For the moment, it is worth saying that studies in imagining machines suggest a soft boundary between the easy and the hard. The easy problem turns out to be harder than Chalmers suggests, while the hard problem may be waning in importance.

Finally, much time has passed since Searle expressed his perfectly justified attacks on the exaggerated claims of the artificial intelligence practitioners of the 1970s. Indeed, in a much more recent publication[4] he clearly suggests that nonbiological machines may be of interest:

> When I say that the brain is a biological organ and consciousness is a biological process, I do not, of course, say or imply that it would be impossible to produce an artificial brain out of nonbiological materials that could also cause and sustain consciousness.

However, he goes on to say that a biological understanding of how the living brain causes mind must be achieved *before* such machines might be designed. I believe this to be an unhelpful constraint. When I say that the heart is like a mechanical pump, I say this because I believe that the heart and the pump have some key principles in common. These principles are reached through an understanding of both the biological and the mechanical at the same time. The great advantage of doing both is that principles in mechanics may not be so well known to biologists, and vice versa. In this book I play the roles of the naive neurobiologist and the naive philosopher but also of someone who brings an advancing knowledge of brainlike machinery into the argument.

My agenda is to show in the simplest possible way that attempting to design such nonbiological systems gives us some additional understanding of how any machinery, biological or otherwise, can sustain conscious imagination and in this way takes us forward in attempting to answer the key question posed above. I do this without losing sight of the fact that the two will always be different: the living brain will have a consciousness that largely reflects its biological nature; the artificially conscious machine will have a consciousness which, by comparison, may be a rum thing, and perhaps may not merit the appellative at all. But it is the mechanism common to the two that constitutes the "additional understanding." While I am not proposing silicon transplants for the brain, I do reflect on the fact that the patient with the plastic heart survives on the basis of the properties common to the biological and the artificial heart. In the same way, I shall be looking at what I know about the artificial that may be common to the real, as we begin the journey toward trying to understand imagination and consciousness.

2

Miletus

Where the Dreaming Begins

The speculations of Thales, Anaximander and Anaximenes are to be regarded as scientific hypotheses. . . . The questions they asked were good questions and their vigor inspired subsequent investigators.
—Bertrand Russell, *A History of Western Philosophy* (1961)

On the Beach

It was a sudden awakening. I had a splitting headache. It looked a bit like the Aegean beach on which I had fallen asleep, except that those who had been with me had now gone. The road behind the beach was still there, but it was cobbled rather than asphalt. The ink-blue Aegean was still there with its wisps of white. Ah, good, I thought; here comes Costa on his donkey. Except that it was not Costa. The donkey rider was very poorly dressed in what looked like an elaborate loincloth. He stopped and addressed me in what was Greek I could just about understand, but not the Greek in which I hoped I would make myself understood. He noticed I was nursing my head and asked if I needed help. "Yes," I said. "In which direction is Eftalou? That's where I fell asleep, I have an awful headache."

"I think you are confused, O Xenon. There is no such place. I think that you must have fallen off a boat during last night's storm, hit your head and got washed ashore. You also speak in a strange tongue. I can only guess at what you are saying. If you like, I can put you on my donkey and take you to my house on the edge of Miletus. Tomorrow you can see a doctor about your headache."

That seemed like a good suggestion, so I got on the donkey, not having allowed the name of where he was taking me to sink in. "My name is Constantinos," he said, "and I am a shepherd, O Xenon." I guess that my name would have been Xenon no matter what I said. It means something like "stranger" I imagined. The name Miletus began to resonate somewhere in the depths of my brain. I knew which was the next question to ask. "What year is it?"

"I am not well versed in such matters and years do not matter to me much, so long as spring follows the winter. But I heard it said that it was the second year after the fifty-ninth Olympiad." (Much, much later, I worked out that it must have been the year 540 B.C.) He led the donkey inland over a hill, and from its brow I could suddenly see a city sprawling among the bends of a river all the way back to the sea. I counted four river harbors full of sailing ships of various sizes. "The river Meander," explained Constantinos, "and this is Miletus."

The resonance grew into recognition: Miletus was the Greek city on the Ionian coast in Asia Minor, often quoted for being the cradle of philosophy. Miletus was occupied and then destroyed by Persians. It was clear to me that these thoughts had to be put aside for the time being. A sense of "oh well, let's see what happens" took hold of my mind.

Evening

Over a delicious fish soup and in the light of a smoky oil lamp, Constantinos felt it necessary to compensate for what he sensed was my total ignorance of the world. He did not want to appear to be harboring a complete ignoramus when the doctor arrived—who, he said, was one of the wisest people in Miletus. Constantinos told me of the disastrous defeat of King Croesus, the wealthy Ionian ruler of Miletus, by the Persian Cyrus only six winters previously and how the

Persian conquerors, having deployed a regime of cruelty and auster-
ity in neighboring Lydia, were now beginning to turn on Miletus.

He remembered former times of great prosperity when Miletus
was trading with far lands through a fleet of sturdy ships, exporting
cloth made from the fleeces of the abundant sheep flocks that were
clearly in evidence during my short donkey trip. Many strangers came
to Miletus so that they could join the trade ships and emigrate to
other lands to start a new life. Constantinos also spoke of earlier turbulent times when power passed from the aristocrats to the cultivators in a bloody revolution, only to be reversed when the aristocrats
gathered their forces again and murdered many cultivators' families.
Things settled down with the spread of the rule of King Croesus,
when aristocrats and cultivators alike learned to benefit from the
material wealth of Miletus. There was a general increase of prosperity, and most lived off the labors of slaves. "But things are so different
now," added Constantinos. "The Persians are treating everyone as
slaves, and," he added as if not to be overheard, "there is revolt in the
air . . ."

He noticed that even though I was an avid listener to his stories
and was asking many questions, my eyelids were beginning to droop.
"Go to sleep now," he said. "Tomorrow you will meet the wise doctor. He will be able to answer some of the questions that I cannot.
Anaximenes is his name."

Morning

"You have awoken early," said Constantinos as he came in from the
yard behind his house with a handful of figs and a leather container
full of sheep's milk. "You seem much better—perhaps you do not
need to see the doctor."

"I would be disappointed not to—I have heard of him," I said, having become genuinely excited at the thought of meeting this figure
whose name again set up a strange resonance at the back of my
mind.

Anaximenes was younger than I had expected—between thirty

and forty, I would have said. But what was striking was his long, prematurely white hair and a strangely wispy white beard. He seemed very fit and there were no signs of overindulgence from food or drink. "Constantinos says that you have a headache and have lost your memory and that you do not know where you come from. You do not look like a Persian—and I hope that you are not as I would refuse to talk to you."

I said that I was not a Persian but could not easily explain where I came from. It was to the north, a place called England. "Then it must be a land near the Euxine sea, so you must come from near the edge of the Earth." Some strange mental link told me that he was talking of what is now the Black Sea—but what's this about the edge of the earth?

"I think that if you keep going north, you reach the North Pole of our globe and not its edge." I was surprised at my own temerity.

"Pole? Pole? Globe?" shouted Anaximenes. "Who has been putting these strange ideas into your head? You must be from Samos. Word has reached my ear that Pythagoras, that attention-seeker, is saying that the Earth is round. Typical! He is always trying to compete with our traditions here in Miletus. But where's the evidence, I ask you?"

I thought it unwise to rise to the question, so I said that I would really like to hear more about the traditions of Miletus. He remembered about my headache and, despite my saying that it was much better, he asked Constantinos to crush some leaves he had brought and made me swallow the juice. It tasted awful.

Why Miletus?

Anaximenes confirmed what Constantinos had said, that since the popular revolutions and counterrevolutions the citizens of Miletus were mainly preoccupied by the wish to get richer. They are all terrified now that Croesus has gone, and the Persians are gradually confiscating everything. I asked whether Miletians had any beliefs in something like a soul or the gods. Anaximenes became pensive and said that, on the whole, people followed what the Orphic priests were saying (less barbaric and more ascetic than the Dionysians, orthodox followers of Bacchus who were given to worshiping intox-ication and enjoyed altered states of consciousness). "The soul is a strange idea and linked with our fear of death. This great sensation of being in the world, enjoying its pleasures, enduring some suffering, loving and hating is our most treasured possession. We know that our bodies decay after death, but we cannot bear to think of the disap-pearance of our feelings of existence. So the Orphics have invented this thought that our internal existence, or soul, transmigrates to another body on death. Each time this happens the soul is purified and eventually becomes at one with God. My own thought diverges from this. It comes from the teachings of Thales, who said that our wisdom must always start with something we can see and fully understand and be developed further by the power of thought itself. We must love the wisdom we thus generate."

I thought, love = *philos* and wisdom = *sophis*. I then asked him to tell me what his conclusions were about the soul. He said that it might be better if he were to tell me first about his two great teach-ers Thales and Anaximander, for it was they who instilled "philosophy" in him, and it is in their ideas that many of his own were born.

The Power of Calculation and Thought

Anaximenes started speaking of Thales and Anaximander in reverent tones and with a tinge of sadness. He felt the need to explain that they had both died a few years before, leaving him to grieve at their departure but to rejoice in the wisdom he had acquired from them.

Thales was a well-traveled Miletian who had been to Egypt where he had learned many rules for measuring distances. He could look up the distance of ships at sea from tables of measurements of their angles from two points on land or the height of buildings from the length of their shadows. He also learned to notice the regularity of the change of position of "moving" stars and came to the notice of the cultivators when he predicted that on a specific day the Sun would become completely darkened.

However, the cultivators and aristocrats alike derided Thales for his poverty even though he had once accumulated some money by predicting a good olive harvest and investing in the ownership of many olive presses in the town. When the rich harvest actually took place, Thales made a profit, but used this more to try to impress on the citizens of Miletus the power of philosophy than to change his own modest lifestyle.

Anaximander was a younger man but was much impressed with Thales's teachings that observation and calculation could lead to predictions that previously had only been the prerogative of priests and oracles. "I remember," said Anaximenes, "when I was not much more than twelve winters old, being allowed to sit quietly in the corner of Thales's house where he was being visited by Anaximander, and the two of them would sit late into the night discussing their agreements and differences about the nature of the world. I can recall many of their conversations, but one in particular stands out in my mind. As you seem to be interested in the soul, I shall tell you of their discussion within the limits of what my memory allows."

Thales's Hypotheses

THALES: My dear fellow, we must yet again start with our point of agreement: the nature of the world and the creatures in it are best understood through our love of a rationally developing discussion rather than the preordained pronouncements of oracles and their attendant priests.

ANAXIMANDER: I have no difficulty in agreeing with this, although I am not so discontent with the assertions of priests. They are using Orpheus as their inspiration for wisdom. His thought has now withstood four hundred or so years of being a multitude of rules whereby men can lead good lives. So when priests tell us of the progressive purification of the soul through its migration at death from the body of one to that of another, this is useful in two ways. First it attempts to explain our feeling of "being," which pervades our waking hours; and, second, it gives it a value, which is diminished by a dishonorable way of using it. For you and me, of course, it poses a completely different question. Is there a soul and, if so, what is it made of?

THALES: Steady on now, my friend. Do I really need to initiate a philosophical investigation into something that a priest uses in order to get people to lead better lives? Why not analyze the benefits of a good life and present these as the right goals for living? The question for us is whether in our discourse about tangible matter—the materials of the world seen and unseen—we arrive at an explanation of our sense of being, at the existence of a soul if you like.

ANAXIMANDER: Nevertheless, there may be something quite clever in what the priests are doing. Their strength comes from their persuasiveness. The story of the migrating soul is appealing and therefore persuasive. If you and I were to declare to the population of Miletus that they should be curious about what their souls are made of, or whether earth, fire, and water are prime substances or not, they would go about their business and ignore us. But when the priests say that if they lead bad lives then their sense of being will be denied eternal bliss, this, they will think, is worth heeding.

THALES: I am not sure that the citizens of Miletus would be interested in any philosophical argument unless it shows them how to increase their wealth.

ANAXIMANDER: My dear colleague, I fear that these musings will not be resolved through our love for wisdom. But I am still puzzling over our more interesting discussions about the prime substance, which over our many meetings have seemed so difficult when thinking of our souls. I certainly cannot see even how we go from any possible observations to working out whether there are souls or not.

THALES: It is important to have hypotheses. These make you think, and even if they are proved to be wrong, that which replaces them leads to an increase in wisdom. My hypothesis about souls is that they are the entity that makes things decide when to move. I notice that while plants and trees move, in the sense that they grow, they need make no decisions because their movements seem to follow directly from the way they are made. But human beings have much choice, and so they have advanced souls. Slugs can also surprise you, although not quite as much as people and so their souls are simpler. I think that all things have a divine content without which they would not exist, gods if you like. But things that choose to move have souls in addition to having gods.

ANAXIMANDER: I need to ask you two questions. The first is how this relates to the idea that water is a prime substance. The prime substance, if I understand you correctly, is then more important than gods or souls.

THALES: This too is a hypothesis, a proposition designed to make you think why it may or may not be true. But hypotheses should never be arbitrary: they must be based in reason stemming from experience. I shall give you my reasons for choosing water as the primary substance and then listen to your arguments against it. The idea is simple, in the world of things capable of dying—that is, losing the receptacle that holds the divine content—the lack of water brings about death. So water is primary because it controls the existence of things whether they have souls or not. It does not affect divinity, and therefore one need not worry as to whether water is more important than a god. Water is the prime substance among palpably earthly substances.

ANAXIMANDER: I shall not dwell on this now, but instead ask my second question. Could *manufactured* objects have a soul?

THALES: Let me think about that—I shall give you a deeper answer some other day, but here is an example that leads me to think that the answer is positive. If I take an iron rod, point it toward the North Star and strike it longitudinally with a rock, I have given it the ability to move toward other metallic objects or cause metallic objects to move toward it. We call it a magnet. To initiate the movement involves a decision as to whether the other object is metallic or not. So, using my movement hypothesis, I would say that in my suggested circumstances a soul exists where one did not before I created the magnet; hence here is at least one man-ufactured object that has a soul. Now, I have been answering your questions. Is it not time that you brought the discussion around to your *own* thoughts?

Anaximander's Theory of Balance

ANAXIMANDER: My thoughts are not as well formulated as yours, but I think of a world of constant change—an evolutionary world where one thing turns into another. For example, where there is fire there will be earth in the form of ashes. There are also changes that must take place over many years: I think that man is a descendant of fishes because he could not have survived with his vulnerable nature until he gradually learned to fend for him-self as fishes do but with greater sophistication.

THALES: Yes, but I thought that you agreed with me about there being a prime substance.

ANAXIMANDER: Indeed I do, but I think that it cannot be water. You see, I think that "balance" is what keeps the world the way it is. I think that all substances have a god who wants to expand his area of influence. Water will put out a fire, but heat will cause water to disappear through drying. So if water were to be the prime sub-stance, its god would have extended its influence infinitely and all but water would perish.

THALES: So which *is* the primary substance?

ANAXIMANDER: Being primary, the substance must be very different from the other competing ones. It is eternal and does not change with time. It transforms regularly into the substances we can per-ceive without altering its ageless and continuous character. In liv-ing things it is the soul, of which we have been speaking; and in all objects it instills a sense of respect for boundaries, which then ensures that the world is not destroyed by the excesses of one entity. The primal substance is in constant motion, so Earth and the stars have been brought into being by this motion and will return whence they came only to be replaced by others, as is the case with objects on Earth. It is this form of justice that gives all things on earth a power to survive in a balanced way and not destroy each other.

THALES: It seems to me that you are putting much more weight on the unknown and the mystical than I would be prepared to do.

ANAXIMANDER: Not really, I just think that my hypothesis is of a different kind: it fits in well with what you have called "reason stemming from experience." My reason tells me that my soul, or the will which lets me decide things, is part of a larger whole. I have difficulties with the idea of migration of the soul, and so an entity that is eternally there but transforms into me—or, eventually, into my successors—seems to be closer to what you were saying about taking responsibility for leading good lives . . .

Anaximenes stopped. "I think that this gives you an idea of how these great minds were engaged in issues that are separate from the concerns of merchants and farmers. In some ways, despite the grief I feel for their deaths, I am glad that they are not here now to witness the total suppression of freedom and justice . . ." His voice began to tremble with emotion and was rising to a falsetto. I thought it necessary to interrupt him. "Tell me more of your own philosophy," I said. "Thales and Anaximander obviously instilled a sense of curiosity in you, and a power to reason."

Anaximenes and Air

"To tell you the honest truth, I found the pronouncements of Anaximander a little too mysterious. He assumed a purposeful life and souls in basic substances, such as air and water, and required them to be just. I find that a little hard to accept, and so my hypothesis is somewhat simpler. I believe that, of the basic substances of earth, air, fire, and water, the primary substance is air; the others appear to me to be condensations of air.

"The first condensation is from air to water—we experience this at night when water appears from pure air. Water, in turn, condenses to form earthlike substances, such as salt at the edge of the sea, and clearly can condense further to form hard substances such as rocks. But the greatest form of air is the soul: it is so clear that I wonder how my mentors missed it! In order to live, we breathe air. If this is made impossible, we die. Therefore the soul, which gives us our sense of being—our ability to decide which actions to take—is made primarily of air. Fire, that powerful substance, I believe to be rarefied air. Air encompasses everything. It makes us alive and surrounds the world and all its beings so as to promote the supporting of life on this wonderful disk we call Earth."

I was about to ask, "What disk? What happens underneath?" when an acrid, pungent smell made my head reel and I must have passed out.

Eftalou

When I came to again, I found that I was propped up under a familiar tree on Eftalou beach with a good old-fashioned bottle of smelling salts under my nose. "This is Dr. Alexi Menos," said Helen. "Costa went to fetch him on his donkey from the village because you seem to have passed out on the beach—I was worried."

"Too much sun," Alexi Menos said. "Sunstroke, you know. Good thing Helen got to you and put you under the tree."

While he was speaking, I noticed his prematurely white hair and wispy beard. The only thing I could think of saying to him was, "You haven't answered my question. What happens underneath?"

Alexi Menos turned knowingly to Helen and said, "Not quite out of the woods yet. He's obviously confused. Perhaps Costa should take him on the donkey over the hill to the house at Molyvos. There he should rest. I'll pass by to see him tomorrow."

"Whatever happens," I thought, "I must remember to thank Costa
for having saved my life—maybe on two occasions . . ."

Ancient Philosophy, Ancient Pitfalls

Very little is known of Thales, Anaximander, and Anaximenes. It is
not recorded whether they talked much to one another, or even
acknowledged each other's existence. I would find it surprising if
they did not, given their likely overlap in time and geography in the
city of Miletus. Certainly, Thales had traveled and gained Babylon-
ian knowledge of geometrical ratios and the presence of cycling in
the motion of the planets. He had predicted the eclipse of 585 B.C.
According to Aristotle, he believed that souls caused motion even
in magnets. And, of course, he appears in the early pages of books
on the history of philosophy for his deductive reasoning that "water
is everything." Anaximander was a rationalist who needed a grander
explanation of the major substances and, uncannily, hit upon the
theory of evolution. However, this need for an ageless overarching
substance led him toward mysticism. Anaximenes returned to the
single substance of air to explain both materialistic and spiritual
matters.

The citizens of Miletus attempted a revolt against the Persians,
but this was brutally suppressed in 494 B.C., when Miletus was
completely destroyed and most of its citizens killed. It is likely that
Anaximenes perished in this destruction. These are the facts, the
rest is an attempt to fill the gaps in some plausible way. There is no
pretense of accuracy; what I have described are just the juxtapositions that dreams are made of.

For me, the reports of the beginnings of philosophy suggest that
the subject itself (love of wisdom) has, from the very start, carried
both inherent pleasures and inherent pitfalls. The pleasures come
from the creation of plausible hypotheses that fit one's personal
experience and deductions. The pitfalls lie, first, in the conflict
between the use of what these days would be called formal methods

(mathematics, physics, etc.) and the acceptance of only those conclusions that are the result of thought and argument. We shall see that the tradition of the great Greek philosophers of the fifth and fourth centuries B.C. (Socrates, Plato, and Aristotle) was to place a great deal of value on their knowledge of mathematics and include this as an element of pure thought. It is not so among philosophers today. I say that this is a conflict because a hypothesis based on careful scientific investigation is most likely to replace an earlier one based on pure thought alone. The Miletian hypotheses about the shape of the Earth are examples of this.

A second inherent problem with philosophy becomes apparent. There is a need for each philosopher to think things through afresh, and he will often wish to deny the thoughts of his predecessors. The idea of consensus becomes unlikely. Even among Miletians it is their disagreements that make interesting reading rather than their agreements. Nonphilosophers have the choice of agreeing or disagreeing with as many viewpoints as there are philosophers. Science, on the other hand, has "paradigms," that is, areas of current consensus and agreement. These paradigms can be overthrown by new findings or better analyses, but they nevertheless help knowledge to progress by directing the work of many toward a common purpose.

Finally, the pitfall of trying to understand "a sense of being," "the soul," or "consciousness" has, right from the beginning, driven philosophers toward mysticism. This was one area where measurements and calculation had to be put aside, and personal beliefs, introspection, and speculation came to the fore. Also, this is the domain of theologians (largely the Orphics in the case of Miletus), and philosophers have to contend with a ready-made theological philosophy that is believed by those around them.

Manufactured Consciousness

It is hardly surprising that the possibility of a conscious machine is anathema to the philosopher: it is a product of calculation and design touching a central issue that philosophers since the days of Miletus have seen as one of the least assailable foci of their deliberations. But, I argue, a conscious machine is a *good* hypothesis for philosophical debate because, at the very least, it demands argued rebuttal. In Thales's imagined words:

> It is important to have hypotheses. These make you think, and even if they are proved to be wrong, that which replaces them leads to an increase in wisdom.

Sadly, many current philosophical rebuttals come from the setting of arbitrary boundaries by dictum. Examples of often heard dicta are: "only living things can be conscious"; "science cannot tackle what we feel inside"; "a mind cannot explain its own existence." Although often well argued, these are but hypotheses possibly waiting to be replaced by others. Still, it is worth remembering Thales's other admonition in my dream: hypotheses should not be arbitrary, but based on personal knowledge and experience. It is more of this that occupies the rest of this book.

3

Nineteen Fifty-eight
A Voyage Toward Interdisciplinarity

There are fields of scientific work . . . which have been explored from the different sides of pure mathematics, statistics, electrical engineering, and neurophysiology; in which every single notion receives a different name from each group. . . . It is these boundary regions of science which offer the richest opportunities to the qualified investigator. They are at the same time the most refractory to the accepted techniques of mass attack and the division of labor. We had dreamed for years of an institution of independent scientists, working together . . . not as subordinates of some great executive officer but joined by the desire, indeed by the spiritual necessity, to understand a region as a whole, and to lend to one another the strength of that understanding.

—Norbert Wiener, *Cybernetics*

There is no subject that I can think of that needs such interdisciplinary effort more than the topic of consciousness. Sadly, this view may not be prevalent among the "great executive officers" of science and engineering of the present day.

—Igor Aleksander

All at Sea: A First Encounter with Wiener's *Cybernetics*

April is an autumn month in South Africa. Days can be warm and sunny or cold and sunny. On this April day of 1958, exceptionally, it was drizzling. I looked over the railing of the m.v. *Jagersfontein* at my parents standing on the quayside. We were all getting wet and pretending to be cheerful. I was the proud possessor of a South African industrial scholarship that would take me to England to study for a Ph.D. with Professor Colin Cherry at Imperial College in London University. I would be back in three years in accordance with the terms of the scholarship.

That was the plot; the subplot in my mind was that I would probably stay in England for the rest of my life. South Africa had not been the happiest of places, and apartheid was something that, living in the country, one could either fight against or ignore, with naught in between. The latter had not been an option for me. I knew that the police had a file on me, as they had for most Witwatersrand University students who were even mildly active protesters. I also wanted to be an engineer. Escape may have been cowardly, but England was a place where active opposition to the foul regime could continue.

I had specially chosen to board the ship in Durban, which added a third week to my journey to Southampton. This was to have been a holiday after what was an intensive four-year undergraduate course in Electrical Engineering: the studying had to be fitted in with the nighttime drum playing in Lyndy's Lively Rhythm Dance Band, and this routine had not left much time for sleep. Unfortunately, in extending the sea voyage, I had not known of my proneness to seasickness, which the ship's doctor attempted to cure with raw herrings. This certainly stopped me from bothering him further, and the problem disappeared once we had rounded the Cape of Good Hope.

As I was leaving South Africa, Uncle Dragutin, who was a qualified mining engineer with a passion for abstract algebra, gave me a book as a present. It was Norbert Wiener's *Cybernetics*. The *dolce far niente* of my period at sea was an ideal time, I thought, to concentrate on this unfolding story of scientists working together to apply engineering principles to an interdisciplinary study of all complex systems, whether they be living or manufactured. I shall return to this theme later, but for the moment I would like to remember Colin Cherry.

Colin Cherry

During my final year studying Electrical Engineering at the University of the Witwatersrand, it was announced that an eminent professor from England was visiting the country. His name was Colin Cherry, the Henry Mark Pease Professor of Communication in the Department of Electrical Engineering at Imperial College in London. He had agreed to give a lecture to the fourth-year students of the Honors course of which I was a member. As far as I knew from my course, "communication" was a subject where one studied valves, amplifiers, the way that electromagnetic waves propagate through space, aerials, and the design of telephone switching exchanges. So I waited for Colin Cherry's lecture with that mixture of resignation ("here's something else to add to the list") and sloppy self-encouragement ("oh well, this is what I've chosen to study, so I may as well listen").

Cherry's lecture was in fact astonishing—no valves, no amplifiers, nor any of the rest. His opening question was whether we knew how bees communicated when one of their scouts had found a pollen-laden flower. There was stunned silence, and so he went on to describe how the scout bee would perform a dance in the shape of a figure-of-eight which had variability in it to enable it to express the direction of the find with respect to the line of the sun. The speed with which the dance was executed was an accurate indication of the distance of the delectable flower. Just as we were wondering what, interesting as it was, this had to do with engineering, he told us in no uncertain terms. Engineering is a process whereby we understand things by designing them. He introduced us to a theory of communication that had been developed by Claude Shannon at the Bell Research Laboratories at Murray Hill, New Jersey. This was intended to measure the amount of information that a communication channel, such as a transmission line, could carry. The theory was so powerful that it could be applied whenever living organisms communicated. With a few simple equations, he completed the argument by working out the number of bits per second that were transacted between the scout bee and the inhabitants of the hive. (A bit is the amount of information contained in the answer to a question in which "yes" and "no" are the only equally likely options. If I ask a friend whether the new baby was a boy, the transaction contains one bit whatever the answer. Had two friends had babies at the same time, the content would be two bits, with which to express, yes—yes, yes—no, no—no, and no—yes.)

Cherry went on to suggest that there were huge questions about how people communicate using language and why it was important for a communication engineer to understand this. Different utterances carry different amounts of information, which can affect the engineering of a system. As communication systems serve mainly to allow people to be in touch with one another, designing such systems without understanding human communication was less than complete.

A Pioneer of Cognitive Psychology

As an example of human prowess that needed engineering analysis, Cherry talked of the Cocktail Party Problem, a phrase with which his name is still associated. The problem is this. Imagine being at a cocktail party and listening to someone's interesting story. This is surrounded by a babble of others telling other stories. It is quite possible for one of these other stories to attract your attention from the one conversation to another: an emotion-laden word such as "murder" or your own name is enough to do it.

Cherry described how psychologists were tackling this problem by doing many experiments that measured which these attention-switching words might be, and by drawing graphs showing the attention-switching probability of different words under different conditions. The power of information theory, he said, was that a more sophisticated model of what might be occurring in the brain (seen as an engineering system) could be derived and understood, and this model was much more revealing than the catalogues of graphs drawn by cognitive psychologists. A "cognitive" psychologist is one whose interest lies in the effect of "thought" on external behavior. This was a relatively new field in the mid-1950s, previous psychology being directed mainly at logging outward behavior and its changes (learning). Two British engineers, Colin Cherry and Donald Broadbent, are classed as occupying a place in the history of psychology as "Britain's pioneer cognitive psychologists" for having added greatly to models of attention.[1] Cherry would have protested at this, as he would rather have been described as a pioneering engineer who had made a contribution to psychology.

As things turned out, I did not study with Cherry. I got to England at the wrong time of the year, and he suggested that a few months in industry before the start of a postgraduate course would be very healthy for me. I stayed in industry for a few enjoyable and instructive years. Among other things, this gave me the excuse for returning my South African scholarship, becoming a British citizen, and removing the need to go back to that troubled country. Professionally, I learned how digital computers were designed and became one of the new breed of engineers called "logic designers." The Ph.D. came later when, in 1961, I returned to the academic world as a lecturer in Communication, first at the West Ham College of Technology and then at Queen Mary College of the University of London. Despite the fact that my thesis was on the design of arithmetic units for computers, Cherry's notion of modeling thought processes was firmly planted in my mind: I would use my newly found interest in digital systems in doing such modeling.

Norbert Wiener and Cybernetic Multidisciplinarity

To tell the truth, I found the on-deck reading of Wiener's book, *Cybernetics*, hard going.[2] The narrative parts were easy to read but so full of diverse facts that it became hard to explain to kind inquirers what the book that I was reading was about. The double integrals in the mathematical center of the book defeated me completely, casting doubt on my freshly acquired idea that maths was a language that I understood. Nevertheless, the way that the book pointed at examples of how mathematics and engineering analysis could unlock some of the major unknowns in the life sciences was a persuasive exhortation to find out more about it. I have reread the book on various occasions during the ensuing forty years and each reading led to a greater appreciation of the deep grasp that Wiener had of a large variety of subjects outside mathematics, from politics to philosophy. On the deck of the *Jagersfontein*, I was just too inexperienced to appreciate it; now I think that it must be one of the most significant science books of the last hundred or so years.

Wiener and his colleagues invented the word *cybernetics* in 1947 and, Wiener writes, it well described the nature of their discussions dating back to the very early 1940s. The group included the physician Arturo Rosenblueth, computer pioneer Vannevar Bush, communications engineer Claude Shannon, neurophysiologist Warren McCulloch, and mathematical logician Walter Pitts. The aim of their discussions was to extend mathematically based scientific methods—that is, the new science of communication and the developing activity of control engineering—to an ever increasing range of disciplines including medicine, neurophysiology, psychology, and even economics. The word *cybernetics* was derived from the Greek κυβερνητησ, meaning "steersman." That is, cybernetics was to be the science of control and communication systems whether they be living, societal, or engineered artifacts.

The world reacted readily to the idea of cybernetics (or maybe just the word). In particular, some business communities and academic social-science departments in universities decided that "a science of communication and control" was just what was wanted to correct the impression that these activities lacked a scientific basis.

I doubt that many subscribed to the furthering of the theoretical side of the subject. Ironically, Norbert Wiener was a man with a deeply felt social conscience. He realized that cybernetics could be used to control and exploit people for the greater glory of company profits. To make his views known on this, he wrote a passionately expressed book, *The Human Use of Human Beings*, which deplored nonegalitarian trends in a capitalist society.[3] This was hardly read, while *Cybernetics* became an international bestseller.

In the United Kingdom in the 1960s, several interdisciplinary undergraduate courses were enthusiastically founded with "cybernetics" in the title. One of these, at the University of Reading, has survived, at least until 1999. But in the world at large, the word *cybernetics* began to be misused. In some parts of Eastern Europe and South America it became synonymous with the application of computers to management. Also, as is often the case with multidisciplinary topics, researchers reverted to the study of the individual topics that made up the compound field. These became called "artificial intelligence," "neural networks," "multivariable control," and "communication systems." Even now, Wiener's identification of the opportunities found at the boundaries of these fields is being largely ignored (with some notable exceptions, such as at the Computation and Neural Science program at the California Institute of Technology).

Some professional societies are trying to keep the spirit of cybernetics alive. I was president of the British Cybernetics Society for a while in the early 1980s, but this was not a happy time. Despite the efforts of a few stalwarts dedicated to the cause (the Society still survives), attempts to return to the rigorous roots of the subject were thwarted by some who wished merely to philosophize in the least rigorous of styles (although this may now have been corrected).

Nevertheless, the cybernetics of the 1940s and 1950s represents a landmark of scientific effort, which anyone wishing to understand and explain the function of living organisms should not ignore. In the rest of this chapter, I shall highlight some of the principles that the pioneer cyberneticians brought to the fore and their relevance more than fifty years later.

Computers and the Nervous System

The early computers known to Wiener were made of electro-mechanical switches called relays. They were used to perform so-called "logical" functions: for example, a relay would act by closing a set of contacts when *all* its electrical inputs were active and be called an AND "gate." Similarly, it could be designed to act when *any one* of its inputs was active and be called an OR gate. Wiener wrote (*Cybernetics*, ch. 5):

> It is a noteworthy fact that the human and animal nervous systems, which are known to be capable of the work of a computation system, contain elements which are ideally suited to act as relays. These elements are the so-called *neurons* or nerve cells. . . . [I]n their ordinary physiological action they conform very nearly to the "all-or-none" principle.

Wiener also drew attention to the fact that his discussion colleagues Warren McCulloch and Walter Pitts were developing electrical-engineering models of these on/off or binary neurons. They showed that the learning that is thought to take place as a result of the variable "strength" of connection between neurons can be represented by a lowly component, as is used in radios and amplifiers: the volume control. Not only does this idea underpin most of what is currently being done under the heading of "neural networks," but it also influenced my own choice of neuron design with which work in machine consciousness is now being pursued (see chapter 5).

Of course, the modeling of coding of signals in the brain and of its detailed structure has now surpassed anything that can be found in Wiener's *Cybernetics*. But what remains astonishing is the insight that he conveys at the "macro" or "system" level of the nervous system; that is, there are principles that stand above the detail of coding and structure, and these were clearly identified at the time. For example, the distinction between long-term memory and short-term memory is explained as an alteration in synaptic strengths (the strengths of connections between neurons, represented as volume controls) for the first, and the ability to sustain a temporary state in closed neural circuits in the second. There is much more of this in chapter 9, where we see that it had taken the best part of forty years for someone (John Hopfield of the California Institute of Technology, among others) to produce an elegant model of the relationship between these two effects. Neuroscientists, however, are generally still much influenced by the McCulloch and Pitts explanation.

Today, computers have achieved prodigious levels of functional sophistication, and one would not wish to express this in terms of the operation of their logical gates. "Word processing," "solving differential equations," or "connecting to the Internet" is more the style of these descriptions. The function of the brain may also be inferred both as we experience it from our own sensations and the way we observe behavior in others. This, too, seems unlikely to be explained by understanding the detailed logical functions of its neurons. But, as we shall see in the chapters that follow, the great fascination in neurocomputation comes from finding methods that express the bulk behavior of a system (i.e., something that makes sense both as a personal sensation and as an observation of behavior). The challenge is to predict this behavior from what is known, which the neurons themselves have learned during a period of education and development. Indeed, Wiener's comment that the nervous system is capable of performing some of the functions of computers is the right way of looking at the computer-brain comparison. It is relatively easy to design a fast calculator that outstrips the arithmetic ability of any human being. But a much more telling, interesting, and important question is how does a human being's brain get to calculate *anything at all*, given its snail-like speed (about a hundred steps per second) compared with that of computers (typically *500,000,000* steps per second at the time of writing).

Feedback: The Essential Ingredient for Thought and Action

Everyone knows about feedback. Whenever someone switches on a public address system and speaks into the microphone, often a dreadful howl is heard. "It's only feedback," someone says, while a technician desperately twiddles the knobs on the amplifier in order to stop it. Sounds from the loudspeakers have got back into the microphone. But why the howl? The closed loop resonates like a vibrating string, the resonance being sustained by the action of the amplifier, a bit like the spring of a grandfather clock that keeps the pendulum swinging.

Wiener realized that this feedback action had a positive effect in living organisms, without which voluntary action could not take place. He gives a simple example of the act of picking up an object with the fingers of one hand. The action involves a large number of muscles. The job of the brain is to control each one of them, but what tells it how much remains to be done? The answer is the distance between where the fingers are and where they should be. This is a combination of what is sensed outside the body, by the eyes perhaps, and inside the body, by the muscles sending signals to the brain about their states of extension or compression. The latter sensing is called *proprioception*. So here is a feedback loop that, rather than howling, performs in a helpful way.

The following little experiment never fails to impress me as evidence of proprioceptive feedback. I hold the index finger of my left hand pointing upwards about 30 cm immediately in front of me. I stretch my right arm hard to the right, out of sight, with the index finger pointing downwards. I make up my mind (?!) to swing the right arm inwards so as to bring its finger as close as possible to the tip of the left finger and to do this as fast as possible. I can do this in a fraction of a second with the accuracy of two or three centimeters. And I can repeat this by starting with my gaze on the out-stretched right hand and the left hand out of sight with little loss in performance. Engineers who design robots and control systems for airplanes have analyzed what is involved in getting this level of performance. It is tricky, and the feedback loop has to be well tuned. Get it wrong in an airplane and there is a danger that the system could start "howling," leading to a crash.

Wiener became interested in whether there were known failures of such systems in living beings. Indeed, he was told of the neurological disorder called ataxia, where in the above experiment there would be a much larger error in the final position of the fingers, and where, therefore, the amplification in the bodily feedback loop is insufficient. Wiener predicted that there must also be occasions where the feedback is too powerful and a "howl" ensues. Indeed, his medical friends told him that such a condition existed, and it is called a "purpose tremor" where, in the above experiment, the right finger would go into a hopeless shaking motion around its target. It is now well known that this is due to hyperactivity of the cerebellum, that part of the brain that controls the muscles that in turn control motion. Suitable drugs can in these circumstances do the work of the technician: they can turn the amplification down (at any rate, for a while).

While the above are examples of human activity that do not involve conscious thought, feedback is ubiquitous in thoughtful activity as well. Fifty years after Wiener's work, in the sort of experiments on artificial visual awareness that we do in my research laboratory, it is our ability to understand the activity of feedback loops that is paramount. The eyes sense and transmit flashes of electrical impulses to many parts of the brain. The brain has to interpret these to decide where to position the eyes next so that the sensation felt by the owner of the brain becomes coherent and complete. But even within the modules of millions of brain cells that make up the many functional areas in this loop, there is local feedback: cells communicate with one another, forming resonating loops, and areas communicate backwards and forwards in purpose-ful ways. There are other loops that cause an organism to predict the result of its actions on the world and that define the very mean-ing of the word *self.* Weiner's insight into voluntary action being impossible without feedback continues to increase in significance as we gain some understanding of the way that awareness—and even consciousness—depend on the feedback loops in the brain.

Communication

As bees help their colonies by communicating the position of the pollen and birds communicate changes of direction in flight to con-trol large flocks, so communication between humans may be seen not just as a way of exchanging pleasantries but as a way of ex-plaining the biological success of human colonies on Earth. More recently, study of communication shows how massive the potential is for expressing observations, ideas, dogmas, philosophies, and the rest in human language. If anything distinguishes the human from the animal, it is this. If anything explains the dominance of the human over physically stronger and more agile living species, it is the power of language. Armed with a theoretical outlook on com-munication, Wiener explored the way in which language creates both cohesion and rifts in society.[4] He warned that the control of communication processes leads to profit, which may not be in the best interest of the society it is meant to serve. He warned, too, of the fact that this puts the control of communication, and hence so-cial cohesion, in the hands of the despot or the seeker of riches. And he pointed out that this then addresses and encourages the parts of society that aspire to power and riches, bringing about a society that tends toward the antidemocratic.

Again, fifty years later, it has become commonplace to apply analysis of communication flows to studies of society. Also, as I write this, I listen to a commentator on the radio talking of the dan-gers of a major newspaper and TV company director's extending his control over the media. But for me, that early insight that communication comes from intentional acts stemming from the "content of our minds" or, indeed, the mechanics of consciousness has been a major driving force in trying to understand how communication modifies the content of mind and how the underpinning neural mechanisms become engaged in doing this.

The Cyberculture

Undoubtedly, *Cybernetics* has had a revolutionary effect on the world of fiction. There are cyborgs, cyberpunks, cyberfreaks, cyberzombies, cyberrats, and countless other horrors. When I talk of making conscious machines, there is a natural assumption that, in common with Dr. Frankenstein, I am about to launch into the world a series of cybercreatures that are bound to have their own evil agenda. I am told that this will, even according to the very principles of Wiener's science of communication and control, cause such monsters to wish at best to enslave human beings or at worst to eliminate them. But this is the stuff of science fiction. In a good sci-fi story, if the cyberzombie does not come close to being an evil force or a superhuman character, the story would not be read. The serious side of thinking of conscious machines is not spectacular enough to find its way into literature.

We shall see that, in order to qualify as a conscious machine, an organism would primarily have the mechanisms of feedback and control that Wiener identified in human beings. But for me, on the deck of the *Jagersfontein*, the effect of this was to plant the seed of the question that still obsesses me: can engineering principles also be applied to the mental side of living organisms? Now, at the turn of the millennium, the positive response I am finding to this question arouses the same excitement that must have arisen among the pioneers of the early days of cybernetics.

For a machine, the mark of consciousness is the ability (possessed by organisms) to know in some detail where it currently is, to understand where it comes from, and to have its own drives to make decisions. It must therefore have a detailed representation of its current position in its world, some knowledge of its own makeup, and a great deal of knowledge about how it might interact with humans. It might be unique among other organisms on Earth in the sense that it could, in principle, communicate with us in our own language. It will understand that, being a machine, it need not compete with us for power, riches, or control.

Fifty years on from the publication of *Cybernetics*, the engineering principles of the nervous system are far better understood. It is also understood that a computer that receives its "intelligence" from a programmer is not an appropriate model for the brain. But the computers anticipated by Wiener, which aim to model the human nervous system (now called "neural" computers), might be appropriate and may well tell us something about our seemingly unreachable minds. But much more of this later.

4

The Ghost of Aristotle

An Influence Across Two Millennia

It is necessary to study [Aristotle] in two ways: with reference to his predecessors, and with reference to his successors. In the former aspect, Aristotle's merits are enormous; in the latter, his demerits are equally enormous. For his demerits, however, his successors are more responsible than he is. . . . [A]fter his death, it was two thousand years before the world produced any philosopher who could be regarded as approximately his equal.

—Bertrand Russell, *A History of Western Philosophy*

After the Lecture

I often lecture on the mechanistic character of the mind. After these lectures, there are many questions. Some are highly skeptical. Yes, the mind of a machine can be defined; but the mind of a living person is sacrosanct, bound up with the (immortal) soul. Or, surely, machines cannot have minds, as these are the (divinely acquired) properties of humans. I usually answer that it is the relationship between the machine "mind" and its mechanics that interests me, because the relationship sheds light on that of the human mind to the living brain. Continuing questions sometimes draw attention to my naïveté for thinking that machines, being man-made, can tell us anything at all about nature-made objects.

The spirit in which these questions are asked suggests that in talking about the minds of machines I am straying outside the boundaries of science and engineering and stumbling into the territory of strongly held beliefs. The audiences to whom I speak are largely Judeo-Christian, and some of the things I say are contrary to many religious beliefs.[1] As a highly lapsed Catholic, I recall my own catechism lessons where "free will" was discussed. I used to ask of my wary teachers of the Marist Brothers order why, given that God wanted us to be good, did he give us free will so that we could do evil? Why did He not give us a will that only allowed us to be good? Why are we more than the products of evolution? The result of this was that I became labeled as a troublemaker in the catechism classes. I also began to feel that in religion there is a way of circumscribing those questions that one can pursue and designating others as heretical even before the answer is found. The latter may not be asked if the answer might threaten belief. Asking questions about the consciousness of machines is one such set of heretical questions. I reacted in life by finding it hard to have a religious belief, but with a passionate interest in where, as a part of our consciousness, such beliefs come from.

Now I realize that Christianity and many of the other contemporary religions are in themselves reflections of much older rebellions against held beliefs. Christianity envelops many ideas that clearly reflect the philosophy of Aristotle, who died 323 years before Christ was born. Judaism crystallized roughly at the time of the Miletian philosophers who, in turn, influenced the "great" Greeks: Socrates, Plato, and Aristotle. Through Christian philosophers such as Saint Augustine and Saint Thomas Aquinas, who were both avid students of Aristotelian philosophy, it is Aristotle who shapes much of Western contemporary cultural beliefs whether or not his philosophy is judged as being sound. It is his ghost who wafts across the podium at question time after the lecture, even if most of the questioners know little of the man apart from having come across his name. But in 324 B.C. Aristotle too was banished, from Athens, accused of having transgressed the boundaries of piety.[2]

Athens, 324 B.C.

Aristotle had freed his slaves, an act that in itself confirmed the suspicions of sensible Athenians, who thought he was so eccentric that he should not be trusted. So he answered the loud knock on the door himself, appearing a slight, scholarly figure to the burly, well-dressed visitor.

"I am Iarchis," said the stranger. "I have some news that you may find distressing." Aristotle gestured to the large man to come in off the street.

"I regret very much to have to tell you that your friend and pupil, Alexander of Macedon, has died," said Iarchis.

Aristotle's face showed the strongest of emotions by not moving a single muscle. "Who succeeded in killing him? He was only thirty-two years old," he said softly.

"Nobody killed him," replied Iarchis. "He died after a short illness in the city of Babylon."

"Thank you for coming to tell me this," said Aristotle, wishing that this obtrusive figure would now go as quickly as possible so that he might compose his thoughts without the outward pretense of being unmoved. But Iarchis remained fixed in his place.

"May I ask who you are?" asked Aristotle. "And is there more that you wish to tell me?" Without asking permission Iarchis, instead of turning to leave, brushed heavily past Aristotle into the sparsely furnished inner room of the house, sat on one of the wooden seats, and beckoned Aristotle to come closer.

"You may have heard of the Hellenic League," said Iarchis, looking up at Aristotle, making him as uncomfortable as possible. "I am an officer of the League. I am responsible for making sure that Athens should not harbor members of the Macedonian Garrison. The hand of Alexander in the government of Athens has never been welcomed by a majority of citizens. His death is welcome, and Macedonians should now leave."

"I am not sure why you are telling me this. My personal knowledge of Alexander goes back more than ten years. I have been an observer of his exploits, as you have been. My concerns are with my school, the Lykeium, where we discuss matters that are above the concerns of either the Macedonian Garrison or the Hellenic League."

"When the Sicilian Euhemeros returned from his travels in Asia with the Macedonian, did he not publish a theory that the Olympian gods who protect us were mere legends?" said Iarchis, attempting to deepen his tone of authority.

"Yes," said Aristotle. "I believe that this was the consequence of his thoughts." Iarchis now stood up, intentionally towering over Aristotle, "Was not your own response one of suggesting that Alexander, as a result of his exploits, had achieved a status greater than these so-called legends?"

"I certainly believe that greatness is achieved through great actions and, to that extent, Alexander has achieved more than any Greek had dared to think might be achieved. This makes him greater than any Greek and hence similar to the Olympic creatures that are thought to be greater than any Greek. I do not necessarily approve of his methods, his cruelty and his disregard of the views of others. I often wonder where these elements of his personality came from. When I was his tutor, we talked of mathematics and logic. He seemed clever enough to solve logical problems, although he argued with me fiercely about pure thought leading to human power. The ability to influence those around him and manage large groups of people seemed to be more important to him. I had not seen him as a great advocate of the power of philosophy. But his exploits have made him exceptional and possibly more important to the citizens of Athens than their legendary gods."

Iarchis again straightened to his full height, "In the League, we have decided that this view requires you to attend a tribunal. You are a Macedonian are you not?"

"I must correct you, I am not a Macedonian. I was born in Stagira in Thrace. I only worked at the court of Macedon when Philip appointed me tutor to Alexander, his son. I do not understand. Are you saying that I should attend a political tribunal for expressing a purely logical point of view?"

"The first meeting will be entirely exploratory: you will be given an opportunity of explaining your position, and we will then decide whether to pursue the charge."

"The charge? What charge?"

"Gross impiety," said Iarchis, sweeping out of the house and leaving Aristotle a concerned and doubly wounded figure. "Alexander, dead . . ." he muttered.

Uncertainty

The date for the preliminary hearing was set. Aristotle was able to think of little else than the fate of Socrates and Plato's account of his trial. Even though this had taken place seventy-five years earlier, Aristotle recognized that he was facing a similar danger. Socrates had been accused of impiety and found guilty of not worshiping the gods whom the state worshiped. And Socrates, thought Aristotle, was a pious man—which he, Aristotle, was not. Socrates went to his death by accusing his accusers of hurting their own beliefs by perpetrating an injustice and so bringing disgrace upon themselves for eternity. They could not hurt him, as his soul would migrate into eternal existence: he was going toward death with pleasure. Even if his beliefs were wrong, he said, death would be a pleasant, dreamless sleep. He refused the alternative to death that was offered to him: the payment of a significant fine. Socrates died thinking that he was merely traveling into an eternal life of pure thought or immortal sleep.

Aristotle felt incapable of such idealism. He saw death as an end to a productive life. His own accusers were devious and would use the charge of impiety as part of their effort to begin cleansing Athens of Macedonians. Aristotle was determined not to give them the pleasure of putting him to death.

He also had grave doubts about the immortality of the soul—or, for that matter, the immortality of any aspect of being a living individual. Inwardly, his thoughts drifted toward his voluminous work on metaphysics, where he attempted to understand the way in which he thought of the objects in the world. He worried about the complexity of his philosophy. With his fate suddenly made uncertain through the visit of the burly Athenian, would there be time to clarify things?

The Soul

His thoughts on the soul had to be made consistent with his ideas about essence: the being of things and the way people talk about them. Things *are* because they contain some material and have a particular shape or function. A tree trunk is made of wood, its "matter," and is recognizable by its shape (its "form"). A ladle has wood in common with the tree trunk, but its shape distinguishes it from the tree trunk. Aristotle stressed that form should not always be understood as visible shape. Form is that which adds meaning to matter. Seen from a distance, a canal and a river could look very similar in matter and shape, but will differ in form merely because the latter is built by humans. Form is what defines the nature of an object, and matter defines that which is necessary in a material sense to give the form its scope. All things have matter and form.

And so it is with the soul. Soul is the form of the body. Soul is that which gives the meaning of "body" to an assembly of flesh and blood components and, as such, it is inextricably linked with the living material of the body. If this material perishes, the soul can no longer act on it and, as a broken vase loses its form, the body becomes a corpse. This, however, does not solve a major conundrum. What kind of a thing is "thinking" or mind? When we see something, what kind of thing is it within ourselves that does the seeing and visualizing (picturing things described by language)? "Mind," taught Aristotle, is that part of the soul enabling the body to think—and in the tradition of Socrates and Plato, Aristotle placed the highest value on the human ability to think. Therefore, if there was anything divine that belonged to a human being in the Aristotelian scheme, it was "mind." It was divine not in the sense of being a gift of God but more in the sense of being an experience during life that is so exalted as to be shared with the highest of beings, that is, whatever Ultimate Creator there may be.

A Tribunal

Aristotle had to wait on a bench outside the House of Justice while the tribunal gathered its thoughts, presumably to work out how they could frame any charges at all. He was clear that its main quarrel with him was that he had served the Macedonian court. The tribunal wanted him out of Athens as a signal to other Macedonians that they were not welcome. And then there was his association with Alexander . . . He vaguely knew Archon, the Prefect of Athens, who was likely to preside over the tribunal. Once, his son had ambitions to enter Aristotle's philosophy academy. Aristotle had judged that he was not sufficiently serious and refused to accept him. This would be remembered.

Aristotle entered the House of Justice and was asked to sit on an uncomfortable stool in the center of the semicircular hall. As his eyes became accustomed to the dim light, he recognized Archon at the center of a group of seven people. Iarchis was seated at his right. Others looked familiar, but he did not know them. Suddenly, he became aware of how he, elderly, balding, with a lisp in his speech, must have seemed to them: a pathetic and defeated figure. Thoughts of pride in his teaching, his voluminous writing, and his confidence in his ability to think lucidly seemed frighteningly inaccessible.

It was Iarchis who opened the proceedings. "Aristotle, you recall having been warned of the accusations that led to the creation of this tribunal: that you place more importance on the achievements of mortals than those of the gods. Do you deny having said that to me?"

"I believe that sophisticated mental acts unite us with the gods. Things I say flow from this belief."

Archon interrupted, "Aristotle, I must warn you, this is not the Lykeium. Do not talk to us assuming that we share your beliefs. We are not gullible students!"

"I know that none of you has been my student," said Aristotle wearily.

Iarchis came back as if attempting to ease the tension. "Our task at the moment is merely to establish whether your continued influence is of value to Athens or whether it is likely to be detrimental to the morals of the young."

"If that is the charge," said Aristotle, finding some force for this exclamation, "I can easily deny it. My aim has always been to raise the ability of the young to think for themselves. If this is a threat to Athens, Athens is in serious danger of becoming a city not suitable for the young at all."

"More pertinent," said Iarchis, "may be the influence you had on one particular individual: the recently perished Macedonian named Alexander. Is he a good example of the benefit of your tuition? Please elaborate on this issue at some length."

Alexander[3]

Aristotle recalled arriving at Philip's court nearly twenty years earlier. He was keen to have this position because, after leaving Plato's Academy, his life had been that of a wanderer. It is true that he married and was deeply devoted to his wife, but he felt the need to settle somewhere and begin giving attention to his own philosophy. His head was full of thoughts that were different from those of Plato, and he wanted to clarify them by writing.

Philip, the King of Macedon, had consulted his physician regarding the education of his son Alexander. The physician recommended Aristotle, who was known to be one of Plato's most brilliant students. He also happened to be the physician's son.

"What was Alexander like at thirteen, when you first met him?" asked Iarchis.

"I was struck by his physical presence. He was what you might call beautiful."

"Did you have or wish to have a physical relationship with him?"

"I see this as a totally improper question. What's more, had you done your investigations thoroughly you would have known how devoted I was to my wife. I am sorry to disappoint you, but if your aim is to get rid of me because I knew Alexander, just do it—but do not use these stupid innuendoes."

Iarchis continued expressionless: "What did you talk about when you first met?"

"Alexander informed me right from the start that he had no intention of accepting a single thing that I would wish to say. I said that I had no particular wish to say anything, but I was willing to hear anything that he would like to tell me. We sat in silence for about half an hour. Eventually he told me that his favorite person was his ancestor Heracles. When I inquired as to why, he answered that it was because he had killed the Nemean lion and then wore his head in battle to intimidate his enemies. I asked him if he too would like to go into battle wearing a lion's head, and he said that he would like that very much. It was clear to me that here was the son of a courageous but ruthless conquering hero, who knew little of the world except the pleasure of conquest and the shame of defeat. In Alexander's world, winning was essential, even if lives had to be sacrificed. We still do not know whether the murder of his father three years later was a plot devised by Alexander's mother. Had she feared that he would take another wife and threaten Alexander's ascendancy? Was Alexander a party to the plot? Sadly, I have observed that Alexander did not value the life of others highly. Perhaps it is some sort of divine retribution that made him die so young."

"What, would you say, was your greatest sphere of influence on the prince?"

"I tried to say something to him about ethics, politics, logic, and metaphysics. He seemed to pay attention only when we discussed the rights and wrongs of going to war. He disagreed violently when I suggested to him that the role of the state was to ensure that status should be awarded according to the level of education of its citizens. He would rather have awarded it for wealth and courage in battle. All in all, in the three years that I spent with him, I formed the opinion that his mind was made up and was no longer flexible. He was not prepared to discuss, listen, or be persuaded when I thought that he was mistaken. By the time he was sixteen and Philip had died, he was ready to assume the role of the conquering king rather than the philosopher king, the latter being the role for which I was preparing him."

Iarchis turned to Archon and suggested a brief break without the presence of Aristotle. When the philosopher had returned to the courtyard outside, Iarchis said to the tribunal, "This is quite hopeless. There is virtually no evidence that Aristotle was in any way significant in encouraging Alexander's ruthlessness. I shall have to change tack and approach the question of his beliefs in divinity."

"Fine," said Archon. "Just get through it quickly. I am getting very bored with this whining man."

A Charge of Impiety

"Aristotle, do you have any respect for divine powers?" Iarchis launched his new attack.

"This is a difficult question to answer, because what you respect as divine power may not be the same as that which I respect. I don't know you, therefore I do not know if you yourself believe in the power of Zeus and the Olympian gods, or the religion of the Thracian Dionysus (or Bacchus, as my father used to call him), or, indeed, the teaching of the followers of Orpheus."

"By the beard of Zeus, Aristotle," groaned Archon, "can you not answer a straight question with a straight answer? Which of these beliefs do you have? Those of Iarchis are beside the point."

"With all respect, Archon, I wish to answer the question so as to make my position perfectly clear to you. I simply wish to establish that beliefs in the Greece of today are not all the same. Mine may be quite different from those of any in this room, but I insist that it is nevertheless my perfect right to hold them."

"Your rights are for us to decide at the moment, so answer the question," said Archon.

"The answer to your question is that I believe in the existence of a God. But this God is not merely a somewhat illustrious human being: He does not even have a human form. My God is not like Zeus or any of the Olympians. The fact that a God exists seems to me evident from the fact that in the world and the heavens we observe objects endowed with motion, and sometimes life. One thing causes another, but something must have been the first cause of all this activity. This entity I call God.

"God is the unmoved mover and needs to be perfect in every way. An object of greatest perfection must be at the source of everything we know. God is that object of ultimate perfection. As, in human beings, perfection is encompassed by the pleasure of pure thought, God exists eternally as pure thought and happiness. He does not, like Zeus and the Olympians, have ambitions or a need for ultimate power. God differs from humans, who have soul and body, by just being pure soul. He is therefore not bound by material matter and is everywhere."

"And how, if I may ask, can poor mortals like me benefit from the existence of this disembodied, all-pervasive, perfect entity? The way you describe Him makes it sound as if such a creature has no bearing on our lives at all, and your belief is therefore tantamount to having no belief at all." This was a new voice.

Aristotle's wonder as to who had spoken was soon resolved by Archon: "Well said, Euripides. Exactly my question." So this was Euripides, the oil and wine merchant who once tried to shut the Lykeium down for discouraging its pupils from getting drunk, as was given to the followers of Dionysus.

"We reach God," said Aristotle, "through the clarity and purity of our thought. That aspiration can be called the love of God. But God has no concern for us in return because He has completed His work in creating our universe."

"Gentlemen, I think that we have heard enough," Archon said in acid tones. "Here we have a man who would, if we believed him, ask us to drop all our existing beliefs in order to worship a ghost who is incapable of doing anything for us. We have, it seems, the grounds for an accusation of impiety. All we need do is set a date for the formal hearing. The result of this, I do not need to remind you, Aristotle, may be that you would be condemned to death."

Aristotle simply left Athens, knowing that all that had happened was part of the beginning of a major purge. He knew that he would not be pursued, as his expulsion was a sufficiently threatening message for the Macedonians left in Athens. He settled in the Macedonian stronghold of Chalkis, where he died a year later, a discouraged figure. It is unlikely that he was aware of the fact that his influence on future thinkers assured for him something close to immortality.

What Has This to Do with Machine Consciousness?

Anyone wishing to check the historical accuracy of the above tribunal need not bother. I claim immunity, as these episodes are the products of my own mind. They are dreams that allow me to visualize what might have happened even when true historical accounts cannot be found. Archon, Iarchis, and Euripides are figures of fiction chosen to fill the yawning gaps in what is known of Aristotle's Athenian trial.

The intended point of all this is that, rather than consider seriously the skepticism greeting the idea of a conscious machine from Judeo-Christian influences, it might be better to go back to the source: Aristotle. Of course, in modern Christianity the influence of Aristotle is felt particularly in the immortal nature of the Christian soul (Csoul), which is akin to the Aristotelian mind (Amind). Interestingly, the Aristotelian soul (Asoul) as the *form* of the body (i.e., that which gives flesh and blood identity) has disappeared from Christian belief. So, how does the suggestion that the mechanisms present in our brains could be mimicked in machines, giving machines something akin to the power of thought, relate to Aristotelian ideas?

The first question is whether the machine has an Asoul. As all objects, according to Aristotle, have form, so any machine has form: this makes it the machine it is. But—and this is the major defining issue—in being the form of a living body, the Asoul defines the living nature of that body. When life stops at death, the Asoul perishes. The word *life* therefore becomes the defining issue, and life here refers to a proper functioning of the biology of the body: heart pumping, liver purifying, lungs breathing, and so on. Most would think of "life" as the property only of a biological organism. A machine (by most definitions that we have today) is devoid of life in the biological sense. Now, according to Aristotle, for an organism to have Amind it must have an Asoul, which clearly would not be available to a machine.

So the questioner who, after my talk of conscious machines, suggests that such talk sounds somewhat heretical has, in some inexpressible way, come to an Aristotelian conclusion. But this realization is helpful because it both holds the answer to the puzzle and indicates that talking of an artificial or nonliving consciousness is worthwhile. First, my sincere questioner has inverted the Aristotelian sequence (life leads in humans to Asoul, which, in turn, has Amind) to a sequence where machine mind (Mmind) implies Asoul implies life. But this is clearly not correct. A machine consciousness (Mmind) implies a Machine form, which implies that it is man-made and devoid of biological life.

Does all this mean that a conscious machine is of no interest at all, and that this book is a great disappointment to all those who were hoping to find a do-it-yourself Frankenstein manual? Certainly, it is my intention to disappoint the Golem makers. But the reason for talking of conscious machines is precisely so as to go beyond the influence of Aristotle and to ask a deep but unoriginal question: How does the Amind arise from the Asoul? In modern terms, what specific properties of the neurochemical makeup of our brains generate our minds? The remainder of the book suggests that the conscious machine gives us some insight—possibly all the insight we need—into what it is that any organism, including the living brain, needs in order to generate a mindlike property for that organism.

5

Early Artificial Neurons and the Beginnings of Artificial Intelligence

In our computing machine technology . . . memories are in frequent use. . . . Pairs of vacuum tubes are mutually gating and controlling each other . . . it is unlikely that the nervous system should use such devices as the main vehicles for its memory requirements.
—John von Neumann, *The Computer and the Brain*[1]

[The brain has] a variety of properties—memory, computation, learning, purposiveness, reliability despite component malfunction—which it might seem difficult to attribute to "mere mechanisms." However, herein lies one important reason for our study: by making mathematical models, we have proved that there exist purely electrochemical mechanisms which have the above properties. In other words, we have helped to "banish the ghost in the machine." We may not yet have modeled the mechanisms that the brain employs, but we have at least modeled possible mechanisms, and that in itself is a great stride forward.
—Michael Arbib, *Brains, Machines, and Mathematics*[2]

Nineteen Sixty-five:
An Interview and Naive Thoughts of Intelligent Machines

The phone call came in the early evening. It was Sir Thomas Creed's secretary. Sir Thomas was the Principal of Queen Mary College where I had applied for a lectureship in the Department of Electrical Engineering.

The interview had been that afternoon, and I had been asked what I would wish to teach and what kind of research might interest me. I said that undergraduate students should know something about the design principles of computers and I would, for the first time in that department, wish to create a course in the theory that this entails. The subject was called Logic Design. I also said—glibly—that in my research I would wish to apply logic design to computers so as to make them much more intelligent than those that were around at the time.

Sir Thomas had looked at me quizzically. "They tell me that this University needs to invest in large computers so that engineers will be able to design airplane engines on them, and that administrators will automate our payroll. As a mere barrister, I find that pretty impressive. They even tell me that one such machine has managed to play a game of chess. But here you are telling me that these amazing machines are somehow flawed, and that you are the person who will improve them."

Incredulity had spread not only all over his face, but had seemed to be driving the sudden changes in the body language of all those around the table. "I need to explain," I said. "I too think that computers are pretty amazing, but they are so different from the human brain. The speed with which a human being can recognize a face or understand the meaning of a sentence seems so far ahead of ways that people are trying to do this sort of thing on computers. The computer has been called an "artificial brain," but it is really just an automated calculating machine. It calculates much better than the brain, but the brain can make sense of the world in which it lives. I want to find out more about the computational mechanisms of the brain, the logic design of the brain, in order to see if this might give us some new ideas on how to design computers."

"What evidence do you have that what you propose is at all possible? How much do you know about the brain?" This had been the only question from the head of the department in which I was to lecture. But it was a killer: I knew nothing about the brain. I had just got a Ph.D. in computer design.

"I know very little about the brain, and I would have to learn. But there is considerable literature published by engineers on models of brain cells and the like. That's where I would start."

On the way home I was sure that I had blown it. Both what I had proposed to teach and what I said I would research must have sounded like badly thought-through ideas. Logic design was taught only in postgraduate courses in other universities, and my intended research must have sounded pretty unrealistic. But having spent four years in developing my Ph.D. thesis on how one can make the arithmetic units of computers go faster, I was pretty fed up with the innards of existing computers. There are no arithmetic circuits in the brain, and yet the brain can do arithmetic. That chain of thought gave me a buzz of excitement. But exactly how I would go about doing anything about it was anything but clear. I was sure that my lack of clarity had sunk my chances of getting the job.

Sir Thomas's secretary, noticing that I had been silent, asked if I could hear her properly. I said that I could. "He would like to offer you the lectureship," she said, and mentioned a salary. "He wants to know how soon you could make a decision."

I had decided many months previously that, if offered the job, I would take it. "I, I . . . er . . . I can make it right now. I am accepting."

"Very well," she said. "When can you start?"

Computers and the Mile End Road

Queen Mary College was architecturally an interesting mix of turn-of-the-century baroque pretense and postwar multistory boxes. Laboratories and offices were efficiently housed. The campus sported a modern chapel and an ancient Jewish cemetery that delineated one of the geographical limits of the expansion of the college in east London. Its surroundings consisted of garages specializing in vehicle bodywork, warehouses specializing in textiles, and hospitals specializing in the casualties of Saturday night excesses.

But I loved it. One often hears the words "academic freedom" spoken as a disapproving mantra, meaning that someone is cutting yet another piece of the higher education budget from educational administrators. While such events are of genuine concern, the feeling that there is freedom in pursuing scientific passions is something quite different from anything else. It is astonishingly pleasurable and gives true meaning to the phrase "academic freedom." My experience so far had only covered the needs of industry and the needs of producing a formal thesis. Certainly, this was not wasted as it helped me get to know what designing computers was all about. But now, in the Mile End Road, I finally felt licensed to ask some scientific or engineering questions to which I would really like to know the answers.

The head of the Electrical Engineering Department was busy selling old computers and buying new ones for the University of London. The demand for computer time by researchers in science and engineering was growing at an alarming rate. One of my fellow Ph.D. students had been persuaded to propose marriage to an operator at the Computer Center, as he thought that this would give his programs some priority. Even so, I think it led to a good marriage!

Three important computer developments were, in the mid-1960s, just beginning to make an appearance. First, it was becoming possible to connect users to large machines through remote Teletype machines. These were like electric typewriters that were able to be connected to large, distant computers over telephone lines. Every keystroke on the Teletype would be transmitted to the computer, sent back and printed on an unwinding roll of paper to make sure that it had not been corrupted in transmission. The second development was the invention of "on-line" computer languages (such as BASIC). These differed from more conventional languages (such as FORTRAN) where the whole program had to be written out and recorded on punched paper-tape and handed to a computer operator for input. Most programs would come back from the computing service with no result, just an indication of errors that may have been committed in preparing them. In contrast, the on-line language could check (via the Teletype) the program as it was being written. Then, once properly corrected, the results would be printed out on the roll of paper only a few minutes after having been submitted to the computer: no operators, no proposals of marriage.

A third development was that of the minicomputer. Digital Equipment Corporation had started making computers that were about the size of a suitcase. The model was the celebrated PDP-8. The price was such that most research laboratories could buy these things. The result of all this was that computers were becoming much more accessible and useful. The case for thinking of brainlike alternatives seemed to be becoming less and less necessary. Computer power and availability seemed to exceed all demand, and any imaginable thing could be achieved with what was available. Sir Thomas Creed's skepticism about my proposed research had to be taken very seriously.

The Brain and the Blackwall Tunnel

In the history of British engineering, the Blackwall Tunnel is hailed as a major achievement. Built in 1897 by Sir Alexander Binnie, it was the second tunnel under the Thames in London, the first being the celebrated mid-nineteenth-century rail project of the Brunel family, father and son. The Blackwall Tunnel joins Greenwich on the south bank of the river to Bow on the north. In the mid-1960s, when I had to use it to reach Queen Mary College from my first experiment with large mortgages in Greenwich, it was just a massive traffic jam. The Victorian bends in the tile-clad underwater duct were designed to allow horses and carriages to move freely but were a major challenge for twentieth-century lorries. Still, despite the exhaust fumes penetrating even tightly shut windows, traffic jams can be used to advantage. A gear change now and then, a brief release of the clutch, and a gentle tap on the accelerator leaves much free time to think. To think about computers. Were they like brains?

The digital computer of the early 1940s was merely an electronic calculator to which the ability was added to store series of numbers. Say that the operator wanted to add up a list of numbers. He would first place the numbers in electronic "registers" (a row of thermionic valves or vacuum tubes, each of which could be on or off). This "memory" of numbers was achieved by encoding the numbers into binary code and switching the valves of the register on and off accordingly. The numbers would be transmitted one by one to the electronic arithmetic unit set to "add," and the sum would appear in a special register called an accumulator. At the end of the operation, the operator would look at the result stored in the accumulator, translate it into normal numbers, and write it down somewhere.

The American mathematician John von Neumann is often hailed as the "father of the modern computer." His ingenious realization was that the actions of the human being in our example above could themselves be stored as codes and held in registers in exactly the same way as the lists of numbers. This special list was subsequently called a "program." It was 1947 and the first "stored-program" computer, the EDVAC, was presented to the world as an "electronic brain."

Computers got faster and more efficient in the intervening twenty years, but their basic principles of operation did not change much. What *did* change was the ease with which they could be used. Computer languages were the heroes of this story. First, in the mid-1950s, came the "autocodes" or "assembly codes" that allowed the operator to give names to registers and memory locations and use mnemonics for operations. For example, part of a program would be written as "mov loc3 to regA; add regA to acc . . ." This dreadful mumbo-jumbo was seen at the time as a godsend, because it bore some relation to what was being done: "move the number in location 3 to register A; add the content of register A to the content of the accumulator . . ." The clever move was that the computer itself was used to interpret the mnemonics and turn them into lists of on/off (1/0) states for valves (in fact, semiconductor transistors by the early 1960s).

The major change came with the "high-level" programming language of that period, namely FORTRAN. This language enabled the programmer to detach the program from the mechanics of the machine. "Add A and B" could be written leaving the computer to work out where numbers A and B were to be held in its large memory. Control information could be included such as "Let C be A minus B and end the program if C becomes less than zero." Again, what the "assembly language" programmer used to do was now handed over to the computer itself. The machine would take the FORTRAN statements, "compile" them into assembly-language sequences (checking at the same time that silly errors had not been made in typing out the program). These, in turn, would be translated into the 1's and 0's that the machinery of the computer could "understand."[3]

No wonder that the thing was called an "electronic brain." Progress over the first fifteen or so years of computer design was one of dragging the human tasks done by a programmer into the computer itself, leaving the programmer ever more freedom to write ever more sophisticated programs. And yet, the sophistication was mechanical: fast calculation, storage of great quantities of data, ever more complex formulas. This improving mechanical performance was clearly of great help in science and engineering: it was the ultimate tool for mechanizing calculations that twenty years earlier would have had to have been done by armies of people and therefore were probably not done at all.

So as the daylight at the exit of the tunnel was becoming visible, the issue about computers and brains seemed to be this. The domain of the computer was that of calculation at high speed, while the domain of the brain was everything else: intention, planning, survival, awareness, fast recognition and recall, and so on. There seemed to be nothing in my knowledge of how computers work that told me much about how the brain does what it does. Where are the engineering principles that tell me how the brain does it? The answer to this question, I thought, was my agenda. Pity I had not thought it through before being exposed to Sir Thomas Creed.

The Challenge of Intelligence

It often happens that, as we define and clarify a plan of action for ourselves, an almost casual event destroys the house of cards we have built, and we need to think things through again. Having divided for myself the world of computing into the calculational, which was the role of the machine, and the rest, which was the domain of the brain, an after-lunch conversation in the college's Senior Common Room convinced me that this distinction was inadequate.

She was a young lecturer newly appointed to the Computer Science Department. We were both formulating our research plans, and I was expressing my thoughts of how we know the engineering principles of calculation but not those of thought in the brain. She said, "Well, of course, people are doing more than calculations on computers. Shannon some time ago wrote a program that can play chess against a human player.[4] Would you not see this as an act of thought, an act of intelligence?"

I had heard of such work, but had seen it as an isolated, interesting example of how far one could go with fast calculation. The chess program represented the positions of the pieces on the board as a long list of numbers. A move was programmed as a formula that changed some of the numbers. By designing these formulas carefully, the rules of chess could be stored in the computer. Because, when playing the game, some board positions are more important than others, a system was created that evaluated the lists of position numbers in terms of value to a player. This gave the machine the opportunity to carry out a massive calculation to evaluate the improvement or otherwise in the board positions of all legitimate moves, and to pick one leading to the greatest improvement. This method of calculation was also used to look several steps ahead in the game and anticipate good moves that the *opponent* might take. So was this not an example of how the power of computation could be used to model the thought that is involved in playing chess?

She had just come back from a visit to Stanford University where a young researcher, John McCarthy, had founded what he called an "artificial intelligence" laboratory. He saw that the methods used to process lists of numbers, as in Shannon's chess program, could be made into a general methodology for solving planning and strategy problems. It would lead to special computer languages. One called LISP (LISt Processing) was already on the stocks. Artificial Intelligence laboratories were being developed not only in California but also at MIT on the east coast of the United States and in Edinburgh in the United Kingdom. The activity was being defined as "doing on computers that which, if done by humans, would be said to require intelligence."[5]

Undoubtedly, this was an assault on my distinction between brains and computers. Back to the Blackwall Tunnel for a revision of my research plans.

The Hardware *Does* Matter

I did not know a great deal about the brain. I *did* know, however, that an expert in list processing did not program it. No matter what my brain was doing, it seemed pretty unlikely that it was processing vast lists of numbers in order to perform intelligent tasks. Just to service the act of driving through the Blackwell Tunnel, it seemed to me that something immediate was going on in my brain. My eyes and other senses were picking up visual information and turning it effortlessly first into vague thoughts (do I need to take the brake off?) and then into detailed actions (press the brake pedal, depress the clutch slightly). In this process, my knowledge of my car and driving nevertheless takes over while my brain deals with more important things, such as "shall I cook some pasta for dinner?" or "what is my research agenda?" Of course, a computer scientist might have suggested that list processing was going on in my brain unbeknown to me. In the rest of this book, arguments will appear that much that can be called "unconscious" thought goes on in the brain to support that which is conscious, but there is no way in which it could be described as the list processing of numbers.

I was also aware that there were those who, by modeling the components of the brain, really wanted to know how a bunch of brain cells could *learn* to behave in these intelligent ways. Yes, learning and adaptation seem to constitute one of the dividing lines between list processing and brains. Another seems to be that the brain is a highly structured piece of engineering in which most of what happens is determined by its specialized structure. The engineering of a computer is such as to be as general as possible to let the programmer write his list-processing programs: so, the hardware of the brain *does* matter in letting it do what it does. In the brain it creates specific overall aptitudes, but in computers it is carefully made neutral so as to keep them as general as possible. My agenda seemed to be back on the rails: it's not so much *what* a computer does, impressive or not, but the fact that *how* the brain does something similar is unknown and unlike anything that programmers do under the heading of "artificial intelligence." The brain is efficient, competent, and dependent on an unexplored form of engineering—one inspired (and controlled) by an astonishingly intricate structure or architecture.

In retrospect, we know that thirty years after those trips through the Blackwall Tunnel, the IBM computer Deep Blue beat Gary Kasparov, the then world champion, at chess. Shannon's method had triumphed over the best human player in the world. But attempts by the press to find headlines in the fact that the machine had finally triumphed in intelligence over the human were met by a great public yawn (except among chess players, for whom the way that the computer was programmed to play was of great interest). By the mid-1990s the number of people with some experience of using computers was many orders of magnitude greater than in the 1960s. In the Kasparov defeat they recognized that here was a great triumph for programmers, but not one that may compete with the human intelligence that helps us to lead our lives. After all, trains do not compete with marathon runners; they just get them to the venues where they can do their running.

Neural Engineering

One of the factors that distinguishes engineering from science is that the engineer builds complex systems from simple bits, whereas the scientist breaks complex systems into hopefully comprehensible components. The first is called understanding by synthesis and the second is understanding by analysis. To understand how brains generate mind, or whether artificial brains can have minds at all, I now know that the engineering process and the scientific process need to work in close collaboration. But in the days of trips through the Blackwall Tunnel, it seemed to me important to get to grips, first, with the building brick of the brain: the brain cell, or *neuron*. I should then get to know as quickly as possible what happens when these are grouped together into tiny systems, in particular how "learning" comes about.

Copious literature was available on what neurons do and how artificial versions could be built in electronics. They were kind of, well, "nerdy" would be the modern word. That is, the interest was focused on a novel use of electronics rather than an understanding of the device for what it can do in a larger system. I spent many months in deciding what is the *essential* thing that a neuron does in a system. My reasoning went a little like this. First we accept that neurons communicate with one another. What do they communicate? Putting much detail and many theories (dearly held and fought over) aside, neurons broadcast to many others one of two things: "I am active," or "I am inactive." Many believe that they do more than this. But such beliefs might detract from our ability to understand large and complex brains, while the binary assumption turns out to be most useful in this regard.

Now, a neuron does not just sit there and decide to be active or inactive at odd times. First, there are neurons in our sensory surfaces (for example, the retina in the eye or the cochlea in the ear), which react to events that impinge upon us. The rods and cones in the retina are *transducers* which are fairly well known from elementary anatomy. Cones are neurons that become active if illuminated with light in the wavelength of one of three specific colors, some cones acting on blue, others on green, and a third group on red. The rods come into their own when the light is low and become active at different levels of low light independently of their color. So, taking the activity of all the neurons in the retina, the patterns of such activity are the beginning (only a tiny beginning) of what we call vision.

Then there is the majority of neurons, deeper within the brain. There is a total of one hundred billion neurons (100,000,000,000) within a human, of which only a small proportion are at sensory surfaces. Most of the rest are in the cortex, an area of the brain that is a bit like a sheet one meter square in size but scrunched up to form the outer layer of what is found when the skull is removed to reveal the brain. Parts of the cortex are highly specialized, controlling activity related to color, motion, hearing, language, and so on. The inner neurons each receive a large number (between 5,000 and 20,000) of contacts from other neurons. That is, a neuron becomes active as a result of the pattern of activity of the neurons to which it is connected. But exactly what patterns activate a neuron?

The Neuron: A Tiny Learner

Warren McCulloch and Walter Pitts in the early 1940s had suggested that every contact point (known as a synapse) to a neuron has a weight, or importance factor.[6] So the neuron acts a bit like a good committee, where the chair listens to all the expressed opinions, takes some members of the committee more seriously than others (or assigns weights to them), weighs up all the opinions expressed, and expresses a decision based on all that information. Neural activity appears as a sequence of spike-like electrical impulses at the output of the neuron, the axon. But where does the chair's opinion of members' views come from for each neuron? In most cases it comes as a result of a "learning" period. During this period, the biological chair, by some means or other, is told (by an educator?) what decisions should be made and assigns high weights to those whose input coincides with the desired decision and low weights to those who are providing contrary advice.

The model suggested by McCulloch and Pitts is that, electronically, opinions or activity could be represented by the presence of an electrical quantity (say ten volts). Then any variation in "weightings" could be represented by a volume control: full on and ten volts would reach the neural "chair," whereas at the other extreme no influence would occur. In McCulloch and Pitts's model, the "chair" can then be replaced by a simple gadget that adds up all the received voltages, and if this sum is large enough (say half the maximum), it acts by broadcasting its ten volts onwards.

A university researcher does not have many flashes of insight during a working life, but what seemed to be one for me was the result of my brain-computer worries in the Blackwall Tunnel and an increasing understanding of what a neuron does. The volume-control-plus-adding-gadget model seemed to be expressed in the wrong language: the language of electronic, or "analog," circuitry. It would be more helpful in the brain-computer puzzle to express the work of a neuron in computational, or "digital," terms. What the neuron does at its outer contacts (act/not act) is roughly digital anyway, and so trying to describe what goes on inside in the analog language of voltages and volume controls seemed to me to be a hindrance to understanding how large assemblies of these things work.

I was certainly not the first to think this. John von Neumann suggested in the 1940s that the neuron was to the brain what a "logic gate" was to a computer. A "logic gate" is a little circuit that acts when all of its inputs are acting (an AND gate); when one or more of its inputs is acting (an OR gate); or when its input is quiet—that is, it does not act when its inputs are acting (a NOT gate). The theory of all this is that *any* digital system can be designed by putting together large numbers of such gates.

But in the depths of the Blackwall Tunnel it occurred to me that even this view was wrong. A neuron does a lot more than just act as a logic gate. The neuron is a tiny computer in its own right. It learns; that is, it has a memory and uses that memory to adjust the relationship between what comes into it and what goes out from it. That is a specification for a *computer*, not a gate. So the great structural difference between the brain and a computer is that the brain can be described as a vast, interconnected network of simple little computers. Toward the end of the 1960s, this opened up an abyss into the unknown: the properties that emerge from large assemblies of very simple computers.

Goodbye, Blackwall Tunnel

In 1968, I was offered a readership at the new University of Kent at Canterbury, together with an opportunity of building a team working on neural engineering. My agenda had solidified. There was a need to make tiny digital neural chips that had their own memory, and to develop a theory that was able to predict what would happen in vast circuits of these microchips. I even managed to get financial support for this work, both from industry and from a major funding source.

The day I set off on my own pilgrimage to Canterbury, a second branch of the Blackwall Tunnel was opened. Traffic jams were reduced and—for a while—almost eliminated. I don't know whether this had a detrimental effect on scientific thinking in the East End of London. I do know that it must have reduced the risk of incipient poisoning from exhaust fumes.

6

Liberating Philosophy
The Empiricists

During the first twenty or thirty years of the eighteenth century [Locke's] Essay and [Newton's] Principia gradually shaded out their Cartesian rivals, and it was in their shade that the next great philosophical movement, idealism, gradually acquired its form and strength.

—Michael Ayres, *Locke: Ideas and Things*

A Pushy Producer

The voice on the phone said, "I am making a film for Channel 4, I wonder if you could help us."

"It depends on what you want to know," I said.

"Well, it's about philosophy, but we want to make it very visual, no talking heads, you know what I mean?"

"Philosophy is all about thoughts and ideas which people talk about . . ."

"Yes, I know all that, but have you not made a conscious machine which we could film? Can we show it saying 'I think therefore I am' "? That would make many philosophical points, would it not?"

"Sorry, I can't help you . . ."

Click went the receiver.

There is no doubt that an increasing number of people know what they know from television and radio. That's no bad thing, but it has positive and negative effects. The upshot of the telephone call is that I began thinking a strange thought. Had there been television in the seventeenth and eighteenth centuries, how would the views of the great thinkers of that time have survived the ambitions of pushy producers? That night, a dream began with the same voice saying, "We would like to go and interview some of these ancient chaps. Descartes was it, or Locke? Could you help to explain to our viewers what they are saying in case it gets too . . . difficult. We also plan to ask them what they think about your ideas of conscious machines . . ."

Program 1: "Descartes's Innate Ideas"

ANCHOR: We are just outside the city of Amsterdam. This is the house of Monsieur René Descartes. He has kindly agreed to be interviewed, but not until later. He is a late riser. In the meantime, I would just like to set the scene this snowy winter of 1646. As his name suggests, Monsieur Descartes is French. Educated by Jesuits, he has had military experience in both the Bavarian and Dutch armies. He is a controversial figure and has been admonished by the University of Leyden and, indeed, the Church on several occasions for expressing heretical thoughts. His support of the views of Galileo nearly had him thrown out of this country. It is said that he has invented a new form of geometry, one in which all points on a piece of rectangular paper are described by how far they are from the bottom left-hand corner of the sheet. Five or so years ago he published his famous *Meditations*, from which his dictum "*Cogito ergo sum*" (I think, therefore I am) has hit the thinking world by storm. It is rumored that he is receiving unpublished communications from Queen Christina of Sweden.

[*The door behind the anchor slowly opens. A short, impressive man appears. He is wearing formal clothes, including a sword. He invites the anchor in. Fade-out and fade-in to a neat interior: A table covered in red velvet and a couple of earth globes are in view. Monsieur Descartes is sitting on a large and throne-like wooden chair uphol-stered in red leather. He understands English but does not speak it. He does not realize that he is being interviewed by people from an-other time. He has been told that they come from another country.]*

ANCHOR: It is kind of you, Sir, to speak to us. As you know, we rep-resent a country where there is much curiosity about how great thinkers like yourself have come to your conclusions.

DESCARTES: So, do they not read books in your country?

ANCHOR: They do indeed, but they do like hearing it from the orig-inators of thoughts. I wonder if we could start with the saying that most have heard of: "I think, therefore I am." Could you develop this for us a little?

DESCARTES: Of course, I have written of this extensively in *Medita-tions* and I am a little wary of making synopses of arguments that I have expressed at length. But it comes from what is, and what is not, truth. In my thoughts I could easily be incorrect in my beliefs and, indeed, I might have doubts about whether I have really ex-perienced something or invented it in my mind. For instance, I can think of a fruit which is half apple and half pear but, while I can-not deny that I am having such a thought, it may not refer to a worldly truth. Ignorance may even lead me to make mistakes in matters that are true in mathematics, such as thinking mistakenly that two plus two is five. There remains, nevertheless, something that I cannot doubt: I would neither think wrongly nor rightly if I did not exist. It must therefore be a truth which is independent of my ability to err that my ability to think is proof of my exis-tence. "I think, therefore I am" must be the most fundamental and unquestionable truth.

ANCHOR: Can you say a little more of the doubtful nature of ideas. Are you saying that mind is just some kind of illusion?

DESCARTES: Mind could be several things: a direct reflection of what our senses tell us, something we invent, or knowledge that is

innate. We cannot trust our senses: they are at times too nebu-
lous. There are far too many ways, for example, of sensing a "bird":
it could be large and swooping down from the sky, or very small
and hopping about on a lawn. The senses merely relay these different things, while the true idea of a "bird" comes from my insight into the nature of things. I could also invent things, like the
apple-pear I spoke of earlier, but this is not true knowledge and
therefore not true mind. The true mind is one with which we are
innately endowed, which gives us knowledge of the world that
goes beyond our sensory power and our invention.

ANCHOR: Where do these innate ideas come from?

DESCARTES: Why, they are the gift of God of course!

ANCHOR: What if I do not believe in God?

DESCARTES: Then you are not only being heretical but also illogical,
not to say perverse. It is an innate idea that all things have a cause,
and the primary cause of all things is a force of perfection that we
call God. As the primary creator, God has made us to appreciate
His and our creation and to appreciate His existence. To do otherwise would have been a less than perfect act, which is inconsistent with the idea of a perfect God. So, not to believe in God requires a denial of the innate knowledge, which we patently have,
of this logical sequence of thought.

ANCHOR: I fully understand that you distinguish innate ideas from perception and invention, but how do these ideas reside within us?

DESCARTES: Mind is not open to immediate influence by all parts of
the body, but only by one small part of the brain. This is the pineal
gland, which is said to be the only part of the brain that contains
the "common" sense, that is, the integration of the five senses. It
is the state of this part of the brain that sends clear signals to the
mind even while the rest of the brain is active in many other ways.

ANCHOR: In the country where we live, there is a scientist who main-
tains that machines can be made with a structure similar to the
brain. He says that in some way they must be conscious, that is,
they have ideas and a mind. What is your comment on this?

DESCARTES: This man must be a heretic. I have argued that it is inescapable that only organisms that can recognize innately that they are created by God can have a true mind. Animals do not have such a privilege, the machine made by your scientist can at best only react to sensory information. It will not have innate ideas. It is just an uninteresting automaton.

* * *

"So what do you think?" It was the pushy producer. "Descartes thinks that you are making uninteresting mindless automata?"

"Of course, Descartes's theory of knowledge as innate ideas," I replied, "has been superseded in philosophy by the empiricists, some of whom you will interview next. It is astonishing, however, how influential Descartes's powerful logic has been. Indeed, many of the objections not only to my work but to that of anyone who claims mind to be the result of the function of brain cells have Cartesian overtones. Roger Penrose for example, an eloquent commentator on consciousness, argues that insight is an aspect of mind which is not available to neurocomputational explanations that tell us how perception and visualization might work in the brain. Where Descartes looked for an unusual part of the brain that contains the innate mind, and in doing so found the pineal gland, in a remarkably similar way Penrose looks for a very specialized part of the brain (the microtubules) as the residence of the insightful mind. The fact that consciousness is somehow detached from the operation of nerve cells is a "dualist" Cartesian notion seen by many as interesting but arbitrary when viewed in the context of the work of those who followed. But, clearly, Descartes's belief in dualism appears to have survived alongside less mystical theories."[1]

Program 2: "Locke, the Philosophical Liberator"

ANCHOR: We are in London, 1691. The power of Parliament has been restored with the joint monarchy of William and Mary. The revolution of 1688 had freed England from royal and religious excesses, so that it is now accepting toleration. John Locke, a physician, has been able to return from his self-imposed exile in Holland and was able to publish his *Essay Concerning Human Understanding* a year or so ago. In the exhilaration of newly found social freedoms, John Locke is said to have liberated philosophy from the constraints of overscholarly and religious influence. He is also said to have helped to liberate the politics of his time with the publication of *Treatises on Government*. We shall be speaking to him in this program.

[*The scene reveals a comfortable interior. The sixty-one-year-old Locke is seated in a leather armchair.*]

ANCHOR: Could you explain why your ideas were threatening to previous political administrations?

LOCKE: You see, despite being enormously influenced by Descartes when I was at Oxford, I now disagree with him fundamentally. The difficulty with believing in innate insight as being the foundation of knowledge and religious belief leads too directly to a justification of a divine right. All that a king has to do is claim that his supremacy is right and innate in order to disregard the ideas of others and the consensus of Parliament. My belief in the development of ideas as something that comes from experience and knowledge of fellow beings is intended to dispel the notion of the divine right of kings and bishops and is of major support for rule by representative consensus.

ANCHOR: Are you saying that Descartes is just mistaken?

LOCKE: No, not at all. In all that I have written, I have tried to show that a complete theory of knowledge can be achieved without evoking the notion of innate ideas. Descartes's philosophy is clear and enormously persuasive. I have merely shown that it is not unique and that it is possible to start with some truths that we can argue are self-evident rather than mystical. I am very impressed with the rigorous way in which Mr. Newton has done this for physical science. I hope to have been similarly rigorous in philosophy.

ANCHOR: What is "an idea"?

LOCKE: There are only two kinds: those that relate directly to our senses, and those that relate to the operations that our minds can carry out on the first kind—objects we perceive and their properties. A white horse, for example, induces in our mind the idea of "whiteness" and "horseness." By comparing horses with (for instance) sheep and cows, we create—using our powers of reflection—a new collective idea of a farm animal. Of course, there is much more to be said about ideas: for example, they could be primary (like "horse"), describing objects that are in the world, or secondary (like "whiteness"), coming from our sensory apparatus.

ANCHOR: Are you a religious person?

LOCKE: Oh, very much so. My reason and my experience tell me that there is a God—that is, a Creator of the world in which I live.

ANCHOR: Would you believe someone who says that a machine could be made that can acquire ideas in the same way as a human being, and therefore that it could have some form of artificial mind?

LOCKE: I can neither believe nor disbelieve this. There is much that we do not know. And one thing we do not know is how "mind" which reflects on ideas—that is, makes a person conscious of ideas—comes about from the motions of our bodily parts. But I see this question as not pertaining to that part of philosophy that I find interesting. It has little to do with pondering the nature of knowledge and understanding.

* * *

"There you go," says the pushy producer. "This fellow tells you that what you're doing is of no importance in philosophy. What do you say to that?"

"Interestingly, I often hear this now," I answer, "but some philosophers aim this criticism not only at *my* work but at anyone who tries to link an introspective knowledge of our mind to the working of our brains. In the case of Locke, this can be fully understood, because he specifically states in his *Essay* that his philosophy (and that of the empiricists who followed him) is not concerned with the "motions of the particles of the brain." Certainly, in Locke's time, any attempt to understand the way the brain works by referring to the "motions" of brain particles (which was the method of Newton's science in the physical world) was doomed to failure.

"But now we have much knowledge of the electrochemical working and anatomy of the brain, and things are therefore different. I do not think that Locke was making the point that a link would never be interesting. He was merely being realistic about the state of knowledge in his era. At the present time, some prefer to impose on themselves ignorance of what is known by saying that it is not important to philosophy. It is also fashionable to say that our knowledge is not sufficiently advanced to tackle these important problems. This is an easy position to hold. Recognizing and understanding what is known is more difficult, particularly if it leads to culturally disquieting conclusions."[2]

Program 3: "The Skepticism of Hume"

ANCHOR: Behind me you can see the imposing facade of Edinburgh's famous Advocates' Library. Edinburgh is at its autumn best. Wet leaves of prodigious colors shimmer in the crisp sunlight of the unusual day without rain. It is the year 1750. We are going in to speak with David Hume, the Keeper of the Library. Last year he published a work entitled *Enquiry Concerning Human Understanding*, which, if taken together with his *Treatise of Human Nature*, is being talked of in philosophical circles as a major review of the theories of ideas held by John Locke, who died forty-six years ago. Of course, Hume, now thirty-nine years of age, is also challenging the philosophy of the sixty-five-year-old Bishop George Berkeley of Dublin, who has drawn attention to the fact that our perceptions are all that we can trust in the existence of matter. That is, our belief in the continued existence of matter should relate to our trust in God.

[*Hume has chosen the main library for his interview. Behind him is a seamless wall of books. He is a large, smiling man who is at that point in his life when an air of confidence and an accompanying tendency to corpulence replaces the awkwardness of youth. He answers questions with a kindly look that bears not the least trace of arrogance.*]

ANCHOR: How much do you agree with John Locke that the mind is an empty slate that becomes filled with ideas?

HUME: Certainly, Mr. Locke's theory of ideas is most persuasive. It is where my thoughts on the nature of mind started. I do believe that the raw material of our thoughts, or our beliefs, come from experience. I have noted, however, that the impression something makes on me on first encounter is related to, but more vivid than, the idea that represents it in the end. But what is very important is that we need to distinguish between simple ideas and impressions from complex ideas, which are combinations of simple ideas but which need not exist in the real world. For example, I can have the idea of a flying horse even though I have never seen one. But, this does not detach such a complex idea from reality. It is merely a combination of simple ideas that in themselves are obtained from sensory experience.

ANCHOR: What about abstractions or universal words?

HUME: That, dear sir, is simple. They have no substance outside our experience. If you think of an abstract notion of "cat," you will find yourself unable to think of the abstraction. You think of a specific cat, while happy to represent the fact that you have seen several such similar creatures by using the word "cat."

ANCHOR: So what of more difficult abstract ideas such as the "self"?

HUME: I am sure, sir, that here you are referring to the skepticism I have expressed with some force in my *Treatise*. If I examine closely something I describe as "myself," I do not find an object that represents this word. I stumble instead on some specific perception, or a place where several perceptions appear, then mingle and glide away. We have no idea of the place we call "mind," where such perceptions are, or what they are made of.

ANCHOR: Do you believe in God?

HUME: Whether I do or not hardly matters. But I am critical of those who see God as the prime cause, the first builder of the universe. We cannot know of the cause of things; we only notice conjunctions. We cannot observe that cold weather causes ice; we can only observe that the first precedes the second. The true cause of icing is for the scientist to discover. In view of this, how can we pretend to know the prime cause of all things?

ANCHOR: Do you think that man will ever make a machine that can have ideas as we have?

HUME: In order to do this, man will have to know exactly how our bodily brains generate ideas for us. Nothing in our current sciences tells us this, and I am most doubtful that it can ever do so.

* * *

"Hume is against you too," says the pushy producer. "Why don't you give up?"

"I have enormous respect for Hume," I hasten to say. "Despite his skepticism, he tells it the way he sees it. He is totally clear about the fact that people cannot understand the causes of things without finding scientific links. Of course, with our knowledge now, 250 years later, I believe that many of the pieces of the jigsaw of how the neural activity of the brain relates to our ideas are falling into place.

"Hume's skepticism, however, still persists at the level of whether neural knowledge explains the causes of sensation or not. Nowadays most will accept that particular neural action correlates with thoughts, but do we have the science that links the two? I shall argue that we do, and that machines have their place in providing us with this understanding. It is worth reflecting that Hume would probably have been equally skeptical about heavier-than-air machines being capable of flight."[3]

Program 4: "Kant's Idealism"

ANCHOR: It is 1785. We are in the study of Herr Professor Immanuel Kant. He is now in his early sixties and is enjoying the attention that his book, *The Critique of Pure Reason*, published four years ago, has achieved in universities throughout Europe.

[*Kant appears younger than his years might dictate. He has the fine features of someone not often forced to face the elements. Indeed, he was known to be somewhat oblivious to the political turmoil in which he lived (the Seven Years' War and the French Revolution occurred during his lifetime). He was a committed scholar, having served the academic cause throughout his life.*]

ANCHOR: I understand, Professor, that you believe that, while knowledge does not transcend experience, it contains much of what is primary or *a priori*.

KANT: Yes you are right, you have understood my position. I believe that there are areas of knowledge that, while uncovered by experience, contain fundamental and indisputable truths that exist independently of our experience. (Examples are arithmetic and logic.) I need to explain things a little more.

There are concepts that are self-evident: for example, a yellow flower is a flower. We believe this, as to maintain the opposite would be absurd. I call these analytic ideas. They do not represent what I think is known *a priori*. Propositions that are not analytic are what I call synthetic; that is, they are dependent on experience in some way. The proposition that "yesterday it was raining" depends on what I or someone else sensed. I call this empirical. But now take a child who is given a doll. Then, on being given another doll he is told that he is in possession of two dolls. He soon works out that "twoness" is made up of "oneness" plus "oneness" and that this truth is independent of dolls but applies to all objects. This new insight is not empirical but *a priori*; that is, while the experience with dolls is helpful, its role is to elicit the *a priori* knowledge of counting and quantity.

ANCHOR: Does this not leave a problem? [*Presenting these programs had given the anchor a certain feeling of philosophical confidence.*] Where does this *a priori* knowledge reside? Are you saying, as

Monsieur Descartes did, that some ideas are innate and God-given.

KANT: Certainly not! But your question is most astute because it leads me to that part of the explanation of knowledge of which I am most proud. It is this realization that makes me feel that philosophy will need to change from that which Locke and Hume made it.

ANCHOR: Please go on.

KANT: I must warn you that the arguments are not easy, but the answer to your earlier question as to where *a priori* knowledge resides is "within ourselves: it is a property of our perceptual apparatus." I have written extensive proofs of the way in which space and time are just such intuitions. For example, if we come to conclusions about where things outside ourselves are, our sense of the space in which we place such things is there within us. It must precede our experience, that is, transcend it or, in my terminology, be *a priori*. Similarly, time is something for which we must have an *a priori* intuition in order to be able to experience events in time. In addition, I have defined twelve categories that must be intuited in a similar way: things such as reality, quantity, reciprocity, and so on.

ANCHOR: I suppose that geometry is then simply a set of rules that make explicit these intuitions?

KANT: You have understood what I am saying very well indeed.

ANCHOR: One last question please. Do you think that it will ever be possible to build a machine that has intuitions of space, time, and the twelve categories of which you speak?

KANT: You warned me of this question and I have given it some thought. My answer is negative, but conditionally so. As far as I can see, no machine that we know is capable of anything we could call intuition. Machines transform energy into useful form, as Mr. Newcomen and Mr. Watt have clearly demonstrated. But the cognition of a human being, even though energy is involved in keeping the human alive, is internal and probably not available to a machine.

The reason I say that this is conditional is because some day a theory of the transmission of ideas (rather than of energy) might come about. Then, one should ask again whether a machine could have an intuition of space and time. Who is to know?

* * *

"You just made the last bit up," says the pushy producer. "Kant would have never indulged in unsubstantiated speculation."

"You are probably right," I submit without defending my suggestion. "But the striking thing about Kant is his feeling for the way our 'perceptual apparatus' is responsible for major areas of our reasoning and intuition. We are only now beginning to develop the analysis of our perceptual apparatus and what it would need to be a carrier of *a priori* knowledge. It may be wishful thinking, but I would like to think that Kant would have come to the logical conclusion that the function of our perceptual apparatus would succumb to theoretical analysis in due course. He was not a mystic.[4] Nevertheless I find Kant's notion that our *a priori* sense of space is within us quite astonishing. This is precisely what we shall see can happen in neural machines" [see chapter 12].

A Production Conference

PRODUCER: We have one program left. Do we introduce another philosopher or do we try to summarize what it all means?

IGOR: Certainly, no account of eighteenth-century philosophy would be complete without a mention of Hegel, who was thirty years old at the turn of the century and died in 1831. He brought philosophy full circle into believing again in the Platonic ideal of the purity of thought. This is achieved by the process of examining an idea (thesis) and its opposite (antithesis) in order to formulate a better idea (synthesis). Through this, he saw the Western world moving toward purity of thought, that is, a drift toward unity with God—just the sort of theological link in philosophy that Locke and some of his followers tried to diminish.

PRODUCER: He would not have been keen on conscious machines?

IGOR: Certainly not. He would have had me burned at the stake. But that's no reason for leaving him out. He was enormously influential in the twentieth century: Karl Marx was influenced by Hegel's view of an advancing evolution of ideas; and the American philosopher John Dewey had a notion of the world as evolving toward being "more organic," and this approach is said to be a lingering belief in Hegel. Furthermore, we have left out the Swiss-born French Romantic, Jean-Jacques Rousseau who, while not being greatly interested in the mind, was also influential—not necessarily successfully, as he is said to have inspired Hitler.

PRODUCER: Still, we are not making a program about the history of philosophy. I thought we were looking at the influences of eighteenth-century philosophy on current thinking on the mechanics of mind. How do you sum it up?

* * *

Empiricism: The Future Philosophy?

I awoke with a start. By when did the producer want the last program to be written? It dawned slowly that this was not necessary. Thank goodness, *no* program had to be written. But perhaps it is worth stressing what is the significance to me personally of this impressive period of the history of philosophy. For me, it stresses forcefully that the philosophy of any age is inevitably bound up with what is known as scientific fact, despite the claims of some that the two are separate activities. The extraordinary philosophical developments of the eighteenth century took place against a backdrop of Newton's novel insights into the physical sciences. But as such scientific development took hold, empiricists and their successors realized that "mind" could not be defined in terms of Newtonian ideas. Their only choice was to reason in the absence of science.

This is sometimes seen as having contributed to a parting of the ways for science and philosophy. It is my view that this should not be the case. We now know that there is a science that is not concerned, as Newton was, with matter, particles, heavenly bodies and light, but with the transmission and absorption of knowledge. It is my firm opinion that this view opens an opportunity for philosophy and science to be reunited. It is in this new unified context that eighteenth-century empiricism makes a lot of sense. It is in this context that a consideration of machines as cognizing objects lends a scientific framework to the thoughts of Locke and his followers. Conversely, any information theoretician interested in the mechanics of thought will find in the empiricists a surprising source of inspiration.

7

Canterbury

The First Machines

MIRACLE À CANTERBURY: UNE MACHINE S'EST MISE À PENSER . . .
—Daniel Vincendon, *L'Express*, May 15, 1972

If the meaning of the words "machine" and "think" are to be found by examining how they are commonly used, it is difficult to escape the conclusion that the meaning and the answer to the question "Can machines think?" is to be sought in a statistical survey such as a Gallup poll. But this is absurd . . .

We can only see a short distance ahead, but we can see plenty there that needs to be done.

—Alan Turing, "Computing Machines and Intelligence"[1]

Packing My Bags: 1974

I looked out of the window of my office in the recently built electronics laboratories of the University of Kent. I could see the nicely spaced colleges that had come into being over the previous ten or so years. Beyond this "new" university I could see the flat plains of Kent and the imposing silhouette of Canterbury Cathedral. I had been much involved with the growth of this institution since my arrival in 1968. Then, it had been half the size it had grown to by 1974, and much of it could be reached only by crossing muddy fields. In an unexpected way, helping to create a new university had been exciting and stimulating. There was an encouraging feeling of parallels between building an institution and building new lines of inquiry; this was unifying and liberating. Traditions in research and teaching were being established, while the traditions of the institutions from which the new academics had come were mantles that were rapidly being shed.

I guess that the student riots that were so much a feature of the late sixties were partly due to the feeling that everything was possible. So why not begin building machines that would display cognitive abilities of their own? I mean, abilities to learn and represent the world as it is rather than as interpreted by the stilted and highly constrained methods of artificial intelligence (AI) programming? In the spirit of adventure that Canterbury offered, this was to be my research program.

Looking at the view from my window with the mixed feelings of both excitement at going to new pastures and sadness at leaving Kent University, I was aware that much had happened since my arrival eight years previously. I had built two experimental machines using silicon neurons: "Sophia" and "Minerva." Our silicon neurons turned out to be forerunners of the silicon Random Access Memory (RAM) developed in the United States. The American RAM, with no connection to what we had done, allowed computers to evolve from the air-conditioned giants of the 1960s to the laptops of today. Neural network studies had first developed in the United States in a team led by Frank Rosenblatt of Cornell University. He called his arrangements (very similar to the McCulloch and Pitts arrangement seen in chapter 5) "perceptrons."[2] Then work in the United States had largely come to a halt due to the pronouncements of Marvin Minsky and Seymour Papert at the Massachusetts Institute of Technology (MIT).[3] A trip to this bastion of influence in Cambridge, Massachusetts, had convinced me of the need to understand what happens when neurons interact, because ignorance of this was causing interest in neurocomputational studies of the brain to stagnate. I had also begun to realize that the mathematics of neural networks could be applied to other things in nature. Could, for example, networks of genes be naturally stable without the intervention of evolution? But I am going too fast.

The Silicon Neuron

I understand that the British pioneer of computer design, Tom Kilburn of the University of Manchester, used to tell his students who were getting bogged down in theory, "Go away and make something, even if it is a mistake." Abstract ideas about neurons were all very well, but the time had come to make something. It was clear that physical neural machines would have to be built out of masses of neural cells, but where was I to get them? The idea of setting up a factory-like production line with large numbers of people soldering up the components to make my little electronic neurons did not appeal. But the age of "solid-state circuits" or "silicon microcircuits" was just beginning to appear over the horizon. It was the beginning of thinking in terms of circuitry not as something that needs to be made of components wired together but as monolithic systems carved chemically out of single chips of silicon.

Universities were only studying the processes involved; it was industry where the real production plants for doing such things were being built. Just before coming to Kent in 1968, I had come to an arrangement with a major semiconductor company near the Northamptonshire town of Towcester. In order to support university research, the director of research, Derek Roberts (who was later to become the provost of University College, London) had agreed to make twelve silicon neurons for us. I remember saying to him that what I needed was completely digital, and so, being just a "random access memory" (RAM), this device could be useful in digital equipment not as a neuron but as a little local memory. Roberts laughed at the naïveté of this academic. Had I not thought of the problem that such a memory would be of limited use because, when the power was switched off, it would lose its content? No, he said, real

engineering systems would go on using systems made of little magnetic ferrite rings which did not suffer such indignities. This discussion took place in 1967. In 1969 the Fairchild Company in the
United States patented the silicon RAM. The indignity of losing information? It was resolved by having little batteries in the equipment. RAMs now provide the local storage for every laptop, every
desktop computer, and every mainframe in the world. Industries
have been built around the device, and the world economy shivered
in the early 1990s when a RAM factory in Japan burned down,
threatening an increase in the price of RAM, in turn threatening to
reverse the downward trend in the cost of computing.

Now for a little numerical perspective. There is an awkward relationship between the number of inputs of a RAM/neuron and the
number of bits (binary on-off states) that it needs to store. The latter number defines the silicon area required, and hence the cost of
the chip. So a two-input RAM needs to store 4 bits, three inputs
needs 8 bits, and so on (one storage bit at least is required for every
possible combination of binary pattern on the inputs). Modern
RAMs actually store a "word" for every addressing (input) pattern—conventionally 32 or 64 bits. Advances in silicon technology
have made it possible for me, in 1999, to go into a shop and buy
what is called a 64-megabyte RAM for about the cost of a meal in
a modest restaurant. A "byte" for silly historical reasons is the name
given to 8 bits. So 64 megabytes is 512 million bits. This sounds a
lot, and it's enough to run the average desktop computer for local
operations.[4] But as a neuron it is puny. The awkward mathematical
relationship means that this only models an artificial neuron with
less than 30 inputs. Neurons in the brain have anything between
5,000 and 20,000 inputs (synapses), which, if modeled in my way,
would swallow up all the silicon memory in the world for one neuron. Something was wrong in my thinking there! Later we shall see
how this has changed so that we can now simulate quite sizable
neural systems on ordinary laptops.

Despite all this, I turned up at the University of Kent with what were probably the world's first eighteen silicon neurons (the twelve needed plus six spares), all of three inputs each—that is, some of the world's earliest RAMs of eight bits of storage each.

Sophia

Given the neurons, what kind of a "brain" could we demonstrate? We decided to make a "retina" with an array of twelve (3 × 4) light-sensitive cells that would stay on and light a bulb when on. In this way we could "paint" patterns on this array using a simple pocket torch, the kind that has a very small bulb and can be found on key-rings. We used a pluggable set of connections to the 12 × 3 total of inputs to the neurons, which we also arranged into a 3 × 4 array, each neuron connecting to a light to show whether it was on or off. The whole thing was fixed with monitoring equipment and power supplies into a rack the size of a fridge-freezer. We called it Sophia, somewhat pompously referring to the Greek word meaning "wisdom."

What could be done using Sophia? We tried to recognize patterns with a randomly connected input plugboard. We painted an H on the input and taught the top two rows of the output to shine their lights. We then painted a T on the input and taught the bottom two rows of lights to come on. We then tested the system with distorted T's and H's and found that, by counting the number of lights in the two halves of the output, we could indicate clearly whether the input was more like a T or an H. We could also analyze this mathematically, and hence understand exactly how this system did what it did. Simply, any neuron that was connected to the top two rows of the output stored logical "1"s at addresses that came from sampled H's, neurons connected to the bottom two rows stored "1"s at addresses that came from sampled T's. Of course, contradictions could arise that would lead to errors in the output, but their probability was low, due to the difference between a T and an H, and overall the system would get it right. This first set of results confirmed that this digital arrangement worked in much the same way as Rosenblatt's perceptron, but ours was purely digital whereas the perceptron was analog with variable weights.

Is there an advantage in being digital? Does this not depart from the biological, which is likely not to be digital at all? At the University of Kent, rightly or wrongly I was beginning to develop an attitude to these questions that has remained with me to this day. When modeling neural systems, what matters is the behavior of the net. Each neuron in the net must behave in its essential features of learning and generalization like a real neuron, but only at its outer boundaries. And this, to a first approximation, is digital activity: firing or not firing. This view allows the investigator to ask important questions about the network. How does its shape affect its behavior? How does the size of the neurons influence things? And so on.

A contemporary reader may, however, wonder why we had not done the whole thing by computer simulation. The answer is simple: computer facilities were not up to it. They still worked mainly in "cafeteria" style, where one handed in programs to the computer center on one day and got the answers back the next. So Sophia, as a special-purpose neural system, would allow us to perform in half an hour experiments that would take a week in computer simulation. Now, of course, we do everything by computer simulation.

In the meantime, in the United States the storm clouds of opposition to neural computing were gathering. Marvin Minsky and Seymour Papert at MIT had discovered computations that these pattern-recognition systems could not do. But more of that in a few paragraphs.

Cognition or Recognition?

Had there been a goddess of science looking at the advances of mortals who call themselves scientists or engineers, she would have noticed that things were going wrong in Canterbury. The very first experiment performed on Sophia was the exercise in pattern recognition described above—is it a T or an H? However, one of the stated aims of the research was to reveal something about how the neurons in the brain contribute to our power to think, that is, to our "cognition." Pattern recognition is a process whereby complex data, such as (say) the many ways of writing the letters of the alphabet, is decoded into a simple set of codes that gives only the necessary twenty-six classifications. So a "T" written in Gothic script or a "T" written in Times New Roman would, in a good pattern-recognizer, generate the same code (say a binary sequence such as 01101). All H's would perhaps lead to 00111. As human beings, instead of the letters of the alphabet we may be trying to decide whether the thing before us is a sheep or a wolf. Is it really the case that the two generate different codes in our heads before we decide to turn around and run in one case and not the other? Is there one code for all dangerous animals and another one for all cuddly ones? This is most unlikely.

There is no doubt that neural networks do a good job of pattern recognition, and it is also likely that this property contributes to the functioning of the odd corner of the brain. But the essence of what the brain does is to reflect on what its external senses are providing. Cognition is a matter of inner activity rather than blind reaction to stimuli. The science goddess somehow or other put this worry in my head and, with some of the Kent University students, we designed a new experiment. This was not an experiment with Sophia, but an experiment on visual perception that we would carry out on our colleagues and other students.

Alan Learns to Recognize

Neural pattern-recognition machines need to learn many examples of distorted versions of prototypes before they can recognize other distorted versions. We decided to test human subjects to see how their ability to learn distortions matched some theoretically predicted behavior of neural pattern recognizers. But, of course, we could not use T's and H's because people know them already. So we used the T and H data but camouflaged it in the following way. We painted T's and H's of various shapes (with them still "looking" like T's and H's) on a 16 × 16 binary grid. We then redrew these shapes, using a computer, by randomly shuffling the boxes of the grid around. We used the same reshuffling for all the patterns. So what started off as recognizable T's and H's then looked like collections of unknown patterns (figure 1). We called them "ducks" for original H's and "geese" for original T's. We first showed the audience one of each, telling them which was a duck and which was a goose. Then we asked them to identify a new "testing" pair. We

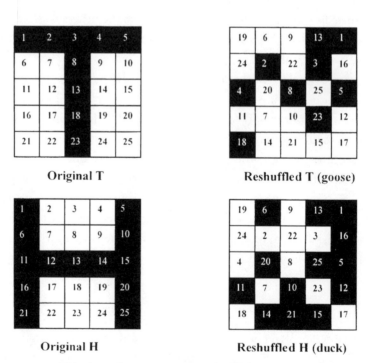

FIGURE I. This shows how a pattern is reshuffled to lose its usual context. Here, 4 × 4 patterns are used, whereas in the experiment described 16 × 16 patterns were studied. The imagined patterns as drawn by Alan were very similar to the reshuffled ones

then named that pair and showed more and more pairs in this way. Indeed, their recognition performance improved like that of a particular neural system with a particular set of properties. But this is not the important result.

On chatting with Alan, one of the "guinea-pig" participants, I asked him to describe why he felt more confident in making his decisions toward the end of the experiment than he did at the beginning. He said that he had worked out what a duck or a goose "looked like." He then compared the new dots in the new tests with his "mental images" and made his decisions that way. To check this, we asked some of the well-performing subjects to sketch out on the 16×16 grid what they thought were prototype ducks and geese. Lo and behold, when we unshuffled these patterns on the computer, the original T's and H's reemerged.

So our subjects did their task by creating a mental image and carrying out "conscious" mental comparisons with incoming sensory data. In contrast, our engineered pattern-recognizers had, to date, no place for mental imagery; it must have made their task more difficult. This exceedingly superficial insight had a profound effect on my work from that moment on. I would need to study neural systems that, as a primary property, would have internal states where mental images (in the case of the visual sense) would be discerned.

It was also the beginning of a niggling worry as to how this inner state in human brains becomes available to the owner of the brain. It was the beginning of what was to become a passionate thirst to find out what was being said by the good and the wise about the neural basis of consciousness.

Sophia and the Inner State

Fortunately, the way we had connected Sophia allowed us to do technical experiments and focus on some theory about inner states. Having a "retina" of twelve picture points (bits) and twelve neuron outputs, the creation of a neural machine with an inner state was easy. We simply connected the outputs to the inputs, and these twelve feedback loops became the site for an inner image for Sophia, rather than something that came in from outside and had to be classified. Now, it was possible to arrange the net so that, painting a T (say) on the input retina would require the network it-self to generate the same T at its output (figure 2). The same could be done for other patterns, each forming, as it were, a pocket of "knowledge" for the net. So the net would build up knowledge with no specific action from a teacher on the individual neurons. In the brain, certainly, no teacher makes specific neurons fire as was re-quired in the earlier experiments on Sophia.

So, in theory, a distorted T coming into the net would be classi-

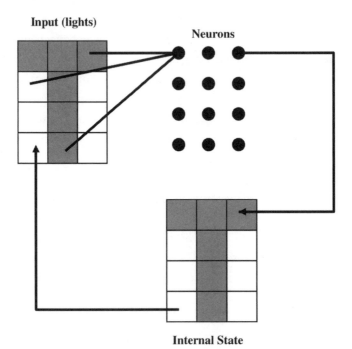

FIGURE 2. The feedback arrangement in Sophia. Only one connection path is shown, but there are similar connections for each neuron.

fied by the fact that the net would internally enter a "prototype" T. But both theory and practice showed that things were not that straightforward. The learned prototype states did not, in those early experiments, remain stable in the net if the net was slightly disturbed. So if the state of the net was T, disrupting just one bit of this state would disturb up to three neurons (connected to the disturbed bit), all of which could disturb the next state in time. This indicated that the net would have to be taught to hold its knowledge even when the input to the neurons was slightly disturbed.

This was 1969 and, many years later in 1982, John Hopfield of the California Institute of Technology helpfully described this kind of behavior in physical terms involving energy. Training on a single T meant that the pattern was like a ball balanced on top of a hill; the slightest disturbance would cause it to fall off. On the other hand, a T learned with variations would, as it were, dig a hole for itself and allow our imaginary ball to remain stable in it. In these terms, our knowledge appears as a landscape full of holes in which the ball of our thought comes roughly to rest when pondering some specific knowledge.

In those early days, we also showed something that would be very important later on: Sophia with output-input feedback would be able to learn to recognize (again by reproducing internally) sequences of input patterns. This is an essential prerequisite of understanding our ability to survive in a dynamic world and to communicate using language.

A Trip to MIT

It was still 1969. A book was sent to me for review from the United States. Its title was *Perceptrons: An Introduction to Computational Geometry* by Marvin Minsky and Seymour Papert of MIT. This was most intriguing as I knew Frank Rosenblatt's book, *Perceptrons: An Introduction to Neurodynamics*, extremely well and wondered how these new authors could get away with a similar headline. I read the book in a very short time and marveled at the mathematical elegance with which they had carried out a serious demolition of Rosenblatt's work by pointing to the computational limitations of these systems. For example, they showed that a perceptron could not distinguish between an odd and an even number of blobs in an image, or classify images according to whether or not they were symmetrical.

The forceful nature of the argument against placing too much hope in neural computation was evident from the fact that the above two tasks can simply be done using conventional computation techniques. The effect of this book on the somewhat small number of people in the United States working on neural systems was phenomenal, and work more or less ceased. Minsky and Papert were warning the world that intelligence could not be modeled from the "bottom up"—or from the neuron up—and that working from intelligent behavior down (top-down) as AI people do was the only way to go.

A closer look in retrospect now reveals that the enthusiasm with which Minsky and Papert were determined to put an end to neural computation led them to being superficial in two areas. First, they had not paid sufficient attention to the power of several neural layers working in cooperation; and, second, they had not thought carefully enough about networks with feedback and internal states. Looking ahead a bit, it was an attack on the first of the two deficits that was the banner of the revolutionary revival in the mid-1980s through the action of what became know as the Parallel Distributed Processing group led by Jay McClelland and Geoff Hinton, then of Carnegie Mellon University, and David Rumelhart of the University of California in San Diego, among many others.[5] The second deficit was rigorously corrected by John Hopfield's papers in the early 1980s.[6] However, by that time many, including my own team, had recognized the power of the inner state and were beginning to be skeptical of the top-down/bottom-up divide. It is the link between the two that needed to be understood.

As the question of the inner state seemed to me at the time to be a serious omission in their work, I decided to visit MIT to thrash out this particular issue. For me personally, the trip to MIT had an unexpected significance.

Minsky in the Cafeteria

I was particularly keyed-up to demonstrate to someone that nets with an inner state (I shall slide into calling the "neural state machines," as we did in our research group) manage to get around some of the problems identified by Minsky and Papert. What I found was that at MIT there was some kind of elation related to the influence of their book on perceptrons, and nobody seemed to be terribly interested in hearing more about it. Mention of neural-state machines got reactions of "Oh, haven't you read the book?" Minsky, despite having himself been a keen contributor to neural networks in his earlier days, was very much involved in setting up "Project Mac," an environment for freely writing and testing AI programs. The AI enterprise was stimulating younger people: Pat Winston and Terry Winograd were deeply concerned with the design of systems that could be said to plan robotic tasks and decipher natural language. Ed Feigenbaum and John McCarthy were developing a strong team at Stanford, and the sense of competition was growing. Everyone seemed relieved by the fact that neural networks had been written off. Why make a computer "learn" when you can write brilliant programs for it?

As these AI systems were being demonstrated, the thought "Is learning not an important element of intelligence?" had to be put aside. Perhaps it was fortunate that, while I was having a hamburger in the MIT campus cafeteria, Marvin Minsky sat next to me and asked me how my meetings with people were progressing. It was then that I said that I felt that something was being missed. Is learning in neural circuits, and the behavior that emerges from this, not important in determining what we call intelligence in the brain? We seem to know nothing about the effect of the structure of networks on their behavior. Is this not an important part of AI?[7]

A Foray into Genetics

Surprisingly, Minsky agreed with me. He asked whether I had, in my visits, spoken to Warren McCulloch. I said that I had not. Warren was ill—terminally ill, as it happened. Clearly, Warren felt the same way as I did. I could, Minsky said, talk with one of the young people in McCulloch's laboratory who was looking at the stability of networks and applying this to genetics. He was Stuart Kauffman who, later in life, was to become an authority on "stability on the edge of chaos." He had simulated networks of two-input neurons, not as neurons but as models of genes. His genes were like my digital neurons but with randomly selected memory content. He took a number of neurons, equivalent to the numbers of genes per biological cell in a particular living species, and interconnected them completely but randomly. So this was clearly a system with internal states and therefore of enormous interest.

What interested Kauffman was the fact that, left alone, these networks would enter a repeated cycle of inner states. Depending on the starting state, differing cycles were entered. Kauffman was able to argue that the number of different cycles found in the net was equivalent to the number of cell types, and the size of the cycles was equivalent to the replication times of these cells. The astonishing property that his results revealed was that, despite all the randomness, the number of cycles and their size was small. This was order where chaos was expected. And the biggest surprise was that this cyclical activity among the states of the net was such that they matched closely with what was found in nature, species for species. This suggested that elements of stability in genetic networks were not due to evolution or divine design but to inherent or emergent properties of the networks themselves.

Sounds complicated? It is. This is not intended as a pun, but this field of research is now known as a branch of complexity theory. Sadly, Kauffman did not have an explanation or a prediction of his results. I returned to Canterbury with a fascinating problem: how could one predict this behavior? These emergent properties were clearly at work, not only in genetic networks but also in all neural state machines, including models of brain activity. Two years later I had published an approximate engineering explanation. The intensity of theoretical work required by this had its toll: a broken marriage and a life led in unheated studio apartments and noisy university residences. Despite this, much of a deep rigorous explanation of order out of chaos remains an open challenge.[8]

Minerva

The obvious sequel to Sophia was a larger machine. An application for funding led to an interview in 1968 by the Automatic Control panel of the Science and Engineering Research Council. I was proposing to use the new neural machine to learn to control robots by modeling the cerebellum, which, in our brains, is very much involved in controlling the movement of our limbs. The chairman, after hearing some of my convoluted arguments for using neural technology, simply asked, "Yes, but what are you hoping to discover which we do not know already?" He was Professor John Coales of Cambridge University, an eminent control engineer. Little did I realize that thirty years later the same research council would have stopped asking this type of terribly important question. It would have asked about how much wealth the research would have created and which commercial company could benefit from it. I answered Professor Coales: "Quite frankly, I am desperately trying to find out how the inner state of a neural network can be controlled during learning. I suppose that I am talking about the "thoughts" that might happen inside this system while it is learning to control the robot. How does a crane driver learn to drive a crane? How does conscious action during learning slip into instinctive activity?

"This sounds more interesting than what we have read in your application," he said, glancing at his committee, "so we had better give you your money. But with your fancy habit of giving these things names, what will you call it?"

Strangely, I had thought about this. "Minerva," I said, very conscious of the fact that this too was pompous in the extreme, "the Roman Goddess of wisdom."

The grant enabled me to commission a small silicon-chip manufacturer to make enough silicon-chip RAMs to make a machine with 1,024 neurons. This machine was linked to a commercial minicomputer—a thing about the size of two large refrigerators. The major task for the machine was to carry out actions that involved internal states. It was demonstrated in 1972 as a device that could learn to control the movement of a simulated vehicle along a simulated road. This is what Daniel Vincendon, a French intellectual, saw when he came to Canterbury with a team from French television. He was impressed, made a film, and wrote an article in *L'Express* that was the first of a series of more than thirty years of press reports that tried to say that here, finally, was the ultimate thinking machine. The fact that research progresses toward goals that are sometimes quite vague and sometimes just passionate curiosities is of no interest to the media. They want to write about breakthroughs.

The Moving Van

The phone call shook me from a dreamlike state, and again I saw the fields of Kent and the cathedral. The moving van sent from Uxbridge was ready; they were waiting for me at my flat at the residences of Brunel University. "We are ready to go, Professor," the voice said. They used my new title, and they came from my new place of work. It sounded strange. I had quite liked being called Doctor.

Yes, during the six years at Kent I had become obsessed with the internal state of neural networks, but I had also grown up a bit. I had seen my first six Ph.D. students through graduation, and some of them were to follow me to Brunel University as staff. I had sent the first draft of my first book (*The Human Machine*, on cognition and machines) to its Swiss publishers. With a colleague, Keith Hanna, I had started writing another one on automaton theory. I had read much about philosophy and psychology and given courses on abstract algebra and logic. I had learned to cook. They were productive years.

Wittgenstein

A Brief Interlude

Extracted from a letter dated March 9, 1930, from Bertrand Russell to G. E. Moore, on reviewing a grant made by Trinity College, Cambridge, to enable Ludwig Wittgenstein to carry on with his researches:

Dear Moore
I do not see how I can refuse to read Wittgenstein's work and make a report on it. At the same time, since it involves arguing with him, you are right, it will require a great deal of work. I do not know anything more fatiguing than disagreeing with him in an argument.
   —Bertrand Russell, *The Autobiography of Bertrand Russell*[1]

A Train Journey to Cambridge

There had been a definite attempt to spruce up the part of King's Cross station where trains leave for Cambridge. I was invited by the Students' Philosophical Society to give a talk at Trinity College on "The Myth of Conscious Machines." I knew that Wittgenstein featured strongly in their debates, and so I was pleased to have recently read Ray Monk's thoughtful biography of this enigmatic man.[2] It was the afternoon return rush from London and I wanted a bit of peace to ruminate over my lecture. I bought a first-class ticket—the students' society would pay the cheaper rate and I would pay the difference, which seemed worth it for the seclusion offered by the little cubby-hole marked "1st."

I was vaguely aware of the yellow brick-clad cutting in which the train was accelerating, with familiar parts of London towering over the top of the cutting walls. Switching my attention back to the compartment, I noticed that another passenger was invading what I thought was my paid-for privacy. It did not take long to recognize the gaunt angular face and the staring eyes: there was no doubt that it was Ludwig Wittgenstein.

Philosophical Interrogations

It took a while to build up the courage, but then I blurted out: "Am I right in thinking that you are Professor Wittgenstein?"

LW: I am certainly Ludwig Wittgenstein, so your thinking appears to be right. Do we know one another at Cambridge?

IA: No, but I am going to Cambridge to give a lecture. I am an engineer from Imperial College in London.

LW: Ah! That soulless place with no philosophy! You know, I too was an engineer once. I did research on kites in the Aeronautics Department at Manchester University. It was a waste of time because the major question for me was why anyone should be interested in kites at all—or, indeed, why anyone should want to do research into anything. The philosophy of science is a grossly underdeveloped subject entirely dominated by adulation for the scientist. I detest the assumption that scientists are neutral in terms of good and evil. Is the atomic bomb a good thing? Is it neutral? And don't tell me that the bomb is the work of those who apply science. It's these arrogant "pure revealers of the truth" who are just as curious to see the effect of the blast as are the engineers and the politicians. The only good thing about an atomic world war would be that it would bring science to an end. So what are you lecturing on?

IA: [cautiously] . . . Computing machinery . . .

LW: I have heard that fellow Turing on the subject. He even asks us to consider that machines could think! That is a very good example of the misuse of words. It is like saying, "I have a toothache," and then setting about discussing the possession of a toothache in the way that you would discuss the possession of a new umbrella. I have read about these powerful calculating machines being called "thinking" machines by ignorant journalists; and then, lo and behold, you get highly intelligent people like Turing wasting their time in trying to work out how machines might think.

IA: I'm afraid that I'm one of those Luddites who ask the same questions.

LW: My dear fellow, how can you be so confused? First of all, we do not know of a machine that can do the job. But worse, it is a nonsensical combination of words. A "thinking machine" is nonsense, like a "flying pig" or a "humorous sky."

IA: What would you say if a machine were to beat a champion at chess. Would that not be "thought" of some kind?

LW: You seem to have some difficulty in taking my point. Of course that is not thought. I would ask where the machine was born, who were its parents and does it appreciate its friends. Don't you understand? To believe that an object can think in the human sense I must simultaneously believe that the object is a human being.

IA: But does one not say that airplanes fly, when two hundred years ago only birds could have been described as flying.

LW: Or kites, indeed! The confusion here comes from the ambiguity of words. A bat is both a flying nocturnal mammal and the thing you swing at a ball in the game of cricket. This does not mean that the two objects have anything to do with one another. So if you chose to call "thinking" what a chess machine does, you are using the word in an ambiguous way. The "thinking" machine and the thinking human have naught to do with one another. The bird and the airplane have nothing to do with one another.

IA: As a former aeronautics expert, would you not say that the bird and the airplane share certain physical properties, such as the aerodynamically shaped wings without which neither could fly.

LW: Yes, indeed. But what an irrelevant argument you are producing. Were I and a sack of potatoes to fall off a high building at the same moment, we would share the force of gravity and reach the ground very much at the same time, but that does not make the sack of potatoes into a philosopher. Sharing the ability to calculate or play chess does not make the computer into a thinking thing.

IA: Turning the question the other way around, does one not talk of living things as "biological machines"? So could one not take their mechanisms and replicate them in a robot?

LW: In describing a person as a biological machine you are describing that person's body. Were you that person and were someone to say to you that your body has a toothache, you would rightly protest that it was you that had the pain. Your body may indeed have a tooth with a cavity, but a cavity and a toothache are not the same thing.

IA: Surely [*I was gaining in confidence*], the cavity and the toothache are but two perspectives on the same event. Without the cavity there would be no toothache, and whatever my pain is, there is something in my body that's causing it. What I am saying is that the cavity is the dentist's only evidence of my pain.

LW: [*beginning to get agitated*] Clearly you have not thought this through. It would be most confusing were we to say that fire and smoke are the same thing because one causes the other.

IA: I must protest, with all due respect. I am specifically not saying that my pain is caused by the cavity, it's just my privileged perspective on the cavity through a sense that the dentist cannot have.

LW: Oh yes? Oh yes? So what happens when the dentist gives you an injection: your pain disappears and the dentist continues to admire your cavity.

IA: But all that has happened is that the dentist has robbed me of my sense. The thing that is common to my pain and the cavity is still there. It is only when the dentist has filled the cavity that the thing (from his perspective) and the pain (from mine) have been removed, even when I get the service of my nerve endings back.

LW: You and I will never agree, because you make the common mistake of believing in some privileged inner perspective. I have long been saying that pains and suchlike, so-called "inner" events, are illusory. Your pain is part of you in the same way as your cavity is another distinct part of you. When you see your nose in the mirror, this reflection is not the same as your nose, neither is it merely another perspective on your nose. Logically it belongs to the set of objects called reflections, a set that steadfastly refuses to admit your nose. I insist that a machine cannot think, as thinking is a word that can only be used to describe what a living object does. It logically belongs to the set of attributes of living objects that steadfastly refuses admission to the things that machines do.

IA: It's worse than that. I shall be asking the students to contemplate "consciousness" in machines.

LW: Heavens above! I spend all this money to get a bit of solitude on this train and what happens? I end up sitting opposite a complete lunatic. The word "consciousness" has a special and unique character. It creates perplexities in our thinking. If I try to answer the question "Am I conscious?," there is a giddy feeling of turning my attention into myself. I find the thought that it is my brain that is producing my consciousness surprising and unclear. I don't understand why I assume that others are conscious. Why cannot I imagine that people around me are automata? All this says to me that the word "consciousness" is some kind of a tool that we use to recognize our own feelings about the perplexing nature of this question. We attribute similar feelings only to others whom we assume to be human. You are asking me to attribute the same thing to a machine that in one fell swoop destroys the normal and fascinating meaning of the word.

IA: I understand what you are saying. Consciousness would not be part of our language were it not for the puzzles it creates for human beings. But is it not the case that scientific investigation changes the meaning of words? For much of history, similar mysteries were assigned to "the heart." It was thought to be the repository of emotions and the focal center of a human being. Now we know that it is an efficient pump. The fact that my brain creates my consciousness I accept as being an idea that cannot be "felt" naturally, in the same way that I cannot feel my heart keeping me alive. I accept that I cannot have insight into the causes of my own consciousness. But just as I feel quite comfortable with the fact that scientific investigation has provided knowledge of how my heart keeps me alive, I would welcome theories of how a brain is involved in consciousness.

You will be pleased to hear that students at Cambridge are great followers of what you are saying. Also, some younger philosophers in the United States, such as David Chalmers (whom you will not have heard of), have taken it further.[3] They suggest that discovering the neural basis of sensation is an "easy" part of the problem and the strange phenomenon of sensation itself is the "hard" part of it. I shall be saying to the students in Cambridge that this is an unnecessary distinction: understanding the former will make the latter less perplexing; therefore, resolving the "easy" will make the "hard" less hard. This modern kind of Cartesian dualism, while appealing, perpetuates the mystique and is unhelpful.

LW: While you are grossly oversimplifying what I have said, I do not altogether disagree with you. In fact, I have gone to a lot of trouble to say that while a statement such as "turning my attention onto my own consciousness" is the queerest thing there could be, I do not see it as being paradoxical. But you must understand that, for a philosopher, the expression "consciousness" is an act of introspection that simply describes his state of attention when he utters the word. An attempt to discuss rather than explain this state becomes his quest. But I do not believe that his philosophical activity will be greatly changed by discussions of the circuits of the brain. So I like what your friend Chalmers is saying.

IA: I think that what you are saying is that a quest to discuss consciousness is a personal matter, not only for each philosopher but also for every human being. This implies that the sense of curiosity for our "sensation" should not be affected by theories based on neural brain activity. This has not been my experience. I think very differently about my own consciousness, having understood what the physical nature of such a phenomenon in a robot might be. That is why I wish to tell the students that thinking of "conscious machines" is helpful in clarifying thinking about conscious human beings. Rather than being a misuse of the word, it is a test of the word—which makes me more comfortable with the word itself when it becomes a state of my thoughts . . .

A train going in the other direction caused a bang and a judder. The carriage became momentarily dark. As the light returned, the person opposite me had vanished. It was fatiguing to try to get my point across, but only because his philosophy—despite being complex—was so persuasive.

9

The WISARD Years

Machines with No Mind

A team at Brunel University, at Uxbridge, near London, has devised a pattern-recognizing computer that, they say, is ten times cheaper than an orthodox one and capable of dealing with jobs as varied as reading addresses on envelopes and spotting flaws in biscuits on a production line.

—Peter Large, *The Micro Revolution*[1]

WISARD (Wilkie, Stonham, and Aleksander Recognition Device) carries out simple processing operations on visual stimuli and succeeds, because of its excellent memory. In contrast, humans show good pattern recognition because of the complex processing of visual stimuli rather than because of the power of their memory systems.

—Michael Eysenck and Mark Keane, *Cognitive Psychology: A Student's Handbook*[2]

WISARD essentially recognizes stimuli by analyzing the statistical properties of two-dimensional images—a solution to the problem of object and face recognition that is probably quite unlike that found in human vision. Nevertheless, by providing an explicit formulation of how face recognition might take place, programs such as WISARD give us a model against which we can contrast and thus learn about human vision.

—Glyn Humphreys and Vicki Bruce, *Visual Cognition*[3]

Uxbridge

Although I had lived in London for ten years before going to Kent, I had never been to Uxbridge. Brunel University was formerly a College of Advanced Technology that had moved to Uxbridge from Acton in the late 1960s. Whereas Acton is a semi-industrial dormitory suburb of London, five or so miles west of the West End, Uxbridge is a warehousing area with a massive Royal Air Force station about seventeen miles west of the West End. Compared with Kent's hillside magnificence, Brunel had a workmanlike gray-concrete appearance among lawns that allowed the wind and the rain to gather accelerated momentum and drench inmates to the bone.

I came to be appointed as Professor of Electronics and Director of Research in the Electrical Engineering Department in 1974 through a curious event. I had actually applied to fill a chair at an old Midlands university. On the train going there, I had bumped into an old friend, Douglas Lewin. Doug was head of the Electrical and Electronic Engineering Department at Brunel. He and I, in different institutions, had been attempting for many years to introduce mathematical methods into the teaching of computer design, which otherwise was a rather empirical pursuit. Doug was finding it difficult to develop his ideas at Brunel, where a somewhat conservative, classical course was being taught. He too had applied for the same Midlands chair. We both needed a position where an advanced and rigorous approach to the analysis of complex digital systems could be established. Needless to say, it rapidly dawned on us that if he and I were to join forces at Brunel, we could create a concentration of expertise in digital systems and develop new courses that recognized the importance of the formal approach to design. The Midlands university had to appoint its third-choice candidate.

I fully understood the implication of this move. Brunel was a place that, named as it was after Britain's greatest engineer of the previous century, had a mission positively focused on the needs of industry. There would be pressure to turn my work on neural machines toward industrial use. This would not be a bad thing, as it would mean getting experience with machine design near the edge of advanced microchip technology and thus developing systems that would not only be competent and useful but could also be powerful enough to begin modeling tiny versions of brainlike systems.

In addition to Doug, there were two other experts in digital systems at Brunel: Gerry Musgrave and Mike Lee. Over the years, the department did become a center of excellence for digital design in the United Kingdom. Colleagues from Kent, namely Manissa Wilson, Ray Glover, and John Stonham, in due course also joined Brunel and worked with me on developing digital neural-network ideas. In particular, John Stonham and I took on a Ph.D. student, the excellent bagpipe player Bruce Wilkie. It is this group that gave rise to the mnemonic WISARD (WIlkie, Stonham, and Aleksander Recognition Device). Completed in 1980, this was the first industrially usable neural-network pattern-recognition machine. Doug left Brunel in 1980, and I became department head as the storm clouds of savage university cuts were beginning to gather. He went to the University of East Anglia, where he founded a new course in Information Systems. Most tragically, he died of a massive heart attack in 1989, soon after his appointment to Sheffield University, where he was about to develop yet another pioneering course on computer design.

The WISARD caught the eye of the press and the media. It was wrongly described as "a machine that recognizes patterns in the same way as the brain." The rest of this chapter explains that this system, though inspired by the brain, owes its success instead to technology.

The Post-Lighthill Era in Artificial Intelligence

My arrival at Brunel occurred at a time in the fortunes of computing that was known as "the post-Lighthill era." This refers to the fact that artificial intelligence in the United Kingdom had been dealt a severe blow. In 1972 an eminent mathematician, Sir James Lighthill, was asked by the Science and Engineering Research Council (the council that funded computer research) to look into progress in AI in the United Kingdom because it was beginning to make great demands on the available budget. His report was damning.[4]

Professor Lighthill suggested that the field was neither throwing fundamental light on the mechanisms of intelligence nor meeting its own targets for useful applications. In particular, he was scathing about a large grant that had been awarded for the design of an intelligent robotic system (Freddy, at the University of Edinburgh) that was meant to assemble a simple toy car. By processing the output of a TV camera, the system was meant to find the parts of the car laid out on a table and devise a strategy for assembling them in the right order. While the AI laboratory concerned had produced a film showing the robot performing a workmanlike task, closer examination revealed some difficulties. The process was much slower than expected and needed to be nudged by a human operator from time to time.

This led Lighthill to spell out what he saw as a major flaw in artificial intelligence methodology, a flaw he dubbed "the combinatorial explosion." AI at that time was deeply reliant on a computer's ability to perform searches among many options in order to find the solution to a problem. Take, for example, a simple stacking problem, where a robot needs to rearrange a stack of three colored cubes (figure 3). Say that the stack starts with a blue block on the table, the red one on top of it, and the yellow one on top of that—expressed as YRB stacked on the table. Say the task is to rearrange this into RBY on the table. The AI system always calculates all the reachable states of the problem. There is only one state that can follow the first one: Y on table and RB on table. And after that there are two reachable states: Y on table, R on table, B on table; or BY on table, R on table.

A human thinker would have the insight to see that the solution can easily be reached in two moves from the first of these states. In

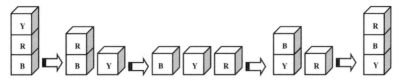

FIGURE 3. Solving the restacking problem.

addition, an observer is likely to formulate a general rule: whatever the initial stack and whatever the number of blocks, any restacking can be achieved by placing the blocks on the table one by one and then restacking them in any required order. The operation would take a number of moves which can be deduced as twice the number of blocks less two. Also, in seeing a stack, a human being can use experience to visualize the solution to the immediate problem with no apparent vast mental search. The observer just "sees" the solution in his or her mind. But at that time, the computer could only solve problems by being programmed to search for a solution among all possible moves.

With three blocks, the set of these new possible states of the problem is relatively constrained, but as the number of blocks grows, the states that have to be searched grows in an alarming fashion (exponentially, mathematicians call it). It is this explosion in the number of states to be searched that defeats the computer in the toy-assembly problem. This led Lighthill to suggest that AI methods were blighted by a "combinatorial explosion."

Paradoxically, I believe that the Lighthill report had a beneficial effect on the world of artificial intelligence, not only in the United Kingdom but the world over. It set programmers thinking of how to make sure that searches of many possibilities had clear constraints on them. It encouraged those who were trying to get the computer to formulate its own rules by examining repeating patterns in the search processes. Furthermore, the clear detachment of AI programs from human ways of thinking about problems was partly remedied by something that became known as the "expert system" or the "knowledge-based system." Here, a human expert's knowledge of something like troubleshooting in motor-car malfunction is "elicited" by a question-and-answer process. A programmer then turns this knowledge into a list of rules. A nonexpert can subsequently use the program and achieve the results of the expert. While this met some of Lighthill's criticisms about a lack of usefulness of AI, it did no more than computerize what would otherwise have been a printed manual.

The early 1980s in the United Kingdom saw a return to optimism through the Alvey program, named after John Alvey, a senior telecommunications engineer with what was to become British Telecom (BT). In the wake of similar "fifth generation" development programs in the United States and Japan, he headed a committee that distributed funds to researchers for developing work in vision, language, and expert systems. Neural-system modeling was not a natural part of this program.[5]

Scene Analysis and an Early Sketch for WISARD

Lighthill pointed out that the way in which AI programmers were proposing to analyze visual scenes also suffered from the combinatorial explosion. The only scenes that were being considered at the time were line drawings of very simple objects such as boxes or wedges. The computer could be programmed to note that particular combinations of lines formed, say, the corner of a box and that specific collections of such corners defined a box. It could then process a line drawing of an assembly of such objects and print out something like "there is a wedge in front of a box." Besides the inability of this method to work with real scenes (involving faces, cows, trees, etc.), Lighthill noted that the number of features such as corners, T-junctions, and L-junctions would grow exponentially with the complexity of the objects and scenes containing them. This is certainly not how people go about recognizing their visual worlds.

The first specification for WISARD therefore was that there

should be no assumption made about the kind of scenes that were to be recognized. It would be a machine that contained as many Random Access Memory neurons as technology and cost would allow. Second, it would have to do whatever it was going to do at the speed that a TV camera generates images. This meant that it would have to do its recognition within one twenty-fifth of a second. Bearing in mind that some classical "line-drawing" recognition programs were taking as long as half an hour to run, there was a clear practical reason for building a WISARD—reasons that might appeal to funding councils.

But life was not to be so easy. The antagonism to neural systems that had started with Minsky and Papert in the United States had arrived in Britain. Many of those who had been deprived of funding as a result of the Lighthill report were not going to tolerate funds being diverted to brain-modeling systems that were "known not to work." So as to build a convincing machine, WISARD would have to be built on a scale unknown in neural work to that date. Sophia (chapter 7) recognized patterns with twelve picture points (3 × 4 arrays) using 8-bit RAM (a total of 96 bits); Minerva (also chapter 7) increased this to 16 × 16 (256) picture points using 16-bit RAM (a total of 4,096 bits), while what was being planned for WISARD was processing 256 × 256 (35,536) picture points using 256-bit RAM neurons (a total of 16,777,216 bits, or 2 megabytes in today's terminology).

Funding councils were not prepared to take this kind of hardware risk and suggested that we should prove the idea by simulation. We had a pretty good state-of-the art laboratory machine at Brunel, but this would allow us to work with only 16 × 16 images with a power of about four Minervas. However, the simulation came up trumps. It was slow, but we were able to demonstrate that some industrial needs could be satisfied. We showed that even with the low resolution of images, the system could learn to recognize pieceparts for real toy cars (we had a little contract from Dinky toys), verify signatures (another contract from Barclays Bank), and sort leather parts cut for shoes (a contract from the British Shoe Association). Despite the protests of the Artificial Intelligentsia, these practical feats eventually persuaded the funding councils to provide the necessary monies for the construction of the WISARD prototype.

And the Philosophy?

Despite its industrial orientation, Brunel University contained a concentration of people who enjoyed discussing the contrast between human and machine abilities. They were in the Cybernetics Department: Frank George and Gordon Pask were great figures in Britain's effort in cybernetics during the 1960s. They were joined by younger people such as Mike Elstob, a physicist/engineer, and David Stewart, a psychologist. One feature of this group was that they held regular Thursday discussions on philosophy—and they invited me to join in. This was a refreshing way of allowing me to stay in touch with deeper issues of machine thought despite the practical turn that my research had taken.

It was at that time that one of the most influential papers in the realm of artificial intelligence was published: John Searle's "Minds, Brains, and Programs."[6] AI experts had been proudly forging ahead with programs that they claimed could understand natural language. Searle used the now celebrated argument of the "Chinese Room" to say that while computers could be programmed to pass comprehension tests on a story that had been fed into them, there was no understanding in their systems. He used the notion of a box that, from the outside, was fed a story in Chinese symbols. It was then fed further symbols that constituted a question about the story. After much buzzing, it would spew out a series of Chinese symbols that correctly answered the question. For example, had the story been about Jack and Jill, the question might have been "Where had Jack and Jill gone?" and the correct answer, namely "Up the hill," would be generated.

Impressive as this might be, Searle revealed that in the box he had placed an Englishman with no knowledge of Chinese, but with a carefully indexed filing cabinet full of rules that told him how to match and process the Chinese symbols. One such rule might be:

> If you see symbols such as "X has gone to Y" in the story, and the question "where has X gone?" then output whatever symbols are in position Y.

Clearly the system needs to have no idea what the objects represented by symbols are like. So, to a question such as "tell me what else you can do with a pail?" it would have to admit that it does not understand the question.

This idea simply planted another question my mind. Clearly, the methods used by AI programmers were being revealed for what they are: symbol manipulation and searching techniques based on rules. But what would stop us from building machines that did have an accessible experience associated with the symbols they use? Maybe they should not use symbols at all, but just have direct inner representations of their experience. The itch to think of designing machines with rich internal states rather than just pattern labels as in WISARD was beginning to make itself felt again.

Personal Constructs

In the spring of 1977 I met Helen Morton, a lecturer in the Psychology Department at Brunel University. A short time later she became my partner.

Helen introduced me to a psychological theory of personality due to George Kelly, an American clinical psychologist. Called Personal Construct Theory (PCT), it seemed to me to be a remarkable view of human thought for the formal way in which it was stated. It has a fundamental postulate and eleven corollaries. George Kelly had been an aeronautics engineer before becoming a psychologist. His key postulate defines the way in which a human being uses his or her experience: by anticipating replications of previously experienced events. Behavior is then determined by a system of bipolar constructs that represent the experience of previous outcomes of taking actions. For example, one of my constructs could be for people on the Helpful-Obstructive dimension. At a party, my behavior would favor talking to those I see as being helpful. At the same party there may be someone with a salient construct in the Exciting-Boring dimension, and she would choose different people to talk to.

The point of all this is that Kelly argued that this system of constructs formed what I would call a "state structure." He also pointed out that these state structures are fairly constrained. They could be elicited formally using a questionnaire, the results of which would form a grid: constructs on one axis, and elements (people, food, career features, etc.) on the other. The boxes would contain an applicability measure. An entire system of therapy had evolved from this idea, and inconsistencies in grids are said to indicate the source of potential psychological problems.

Of all the psychological theories I had known, this had the greatest appeal. It treated the human as being very much an individual—a scientist who not only absorbs passive experience as an internal state structure but, as a living entity, uses this state structure to influence future behavior to continue building the structure itself. All this made enormous sense, not only as a model of traits in the behavior of individuals but also because it included a model of reflective learning as a central part of developing behavior. This was refreshing at a time when computational AI theories of behavior ignored learning altogether. It was also immensely stimulating in making me determined to develop learning systems in which a task for neural networks could be the creation of personality-forming state structures. But, in the meantime, the main concerns remained with the WISARD, which was in the process of being built.

Faces

As the WISARD was being constructed, Adrian Berry, a senior science correspondent of the *Daily Telegraph*, visited the laboratory. A few days earlier there had been a riot at a football game in the Midlands. The question was whether one could build up knowledge in a computer of the faces of reoffending hooligans. Berry asked whether, when completed, WISARD could perform this task. "Definitely not," I said. "The ability to recognize faces is very much wired into primate brains. A general-purpose machine such as WISARD starts from too far behind and would have to learn what is built into the wiring of the brains of human beings."

Bruce Wilkie was there too, and I vaguely remember that he muttered something like "Mmm . . . I'm not so sure . . ." This was one of the few occasions when I have been more cautious in my predictions than one of my students. They normally keep my feet on the ground.

Some months later, Bruce came into my office. "I think that I can demonstrate it working now," he said encouragingly.

"What are you recognizing?" I asked.

"Faces!" was the answer. Indeed, Bruce sat me down in front of the camera and recorded "Hello Igor" in the output circuits of the WISARD and did the same for John Stonham as "Hello John." Subsequently, as we sat down in front of its camera, it would generate the right output even if we changed the positions of our heads, grimaced, or put on a pair of glasses. Someone it didn't "know" would cause a shout of "Intruder!" The powers of its generalization were impressive and the speed at which it made its decisions astonishing.

Most of the time, scientific research looks for a confirmation of theoretical predictions and experiences frustration when this does not happen. This was a very rare experience of genuine surprise because something unexpected was happening. As time went by, we were able to analyze this behavior and show that perhaps face recognition was not that difficult a task. Curiously, as a result of the publicity that surrounded this system, the celebrated Cambridge physiologist Fergus Campbell visited our laboratories. We proudly showed off our input resolution of 256 × 256 picture points and how this could differentiate between faces. "You know," he said, "humans seem to recognize faces presented at very low resolution." In evidence, he reminded us of that famous picture of Abraham Lincoln that can be recognized despite the fact that it is presented on a matrix of only 4 × 5 squares of different shades of gray. All one needs to do to recognize the image is to blur it slightly by half-shutting one's eyes. This removes the effect of the edges of the squares, and up pops Abraham Lincoln.

Campbell suggested that we take down the resolution of WIS-ARD and see how it fares. We went down to 128 × 128—and the performance improved! And so it did all the way down to 16 × 16. At 8 × 8 it collapsed completely—another surprise. "That's all I wanted to see," said Campbell. He explained that in physiology there was a debate going on as to whether or not there were highly specialized circuits in the brain that were supersensitive to differences between faces. The evidence that special parts of the brain react to faces in general was mounting, but taking this to mean that every known face commanded a separate brain area (as some had claimed) seemed spurious to Campbell. Our experiment demonstrated that there was sufficient statistical differentiation between faces to allow a totally nonspecialized neural system to distinguish between them. We subsequently did a lot of work on face recognition for security applications, and in 1982 we demonstrated at the June soirée of the Royal Society that the WISARD could differentiate between smiling and frowning faces, irrespective of whose faces were presented to its eye.

The Commercial World

The WISARD was also shown to work well on many other practical tasks: intruder detection in fields and buildings, banknote verification, packaging control in pharmaceuticals, and so on. The publicity had some curious effects. The Ministry of Defense shut our laboratory down while they considered whether there were defense implications for WISARD. Luckily, they became convinced of its simplicity and that any fool who had read our papers over the last few years would be able to build a similar device. A government agency called the British Technology Group (BTG) insisted on taking out a patent on the university's behalf, despite the fact that a few years earlier they had turned down our application to fund and protect the idea. Their rejection letter had suggested that unproven neural technology could not compete with current artificial intelligence techniques. Now they were threatening exorbitant licensing rates for anyone who would wish to use the patent, and totally failed to interest anyone. This caught the attention of an old friend, computer vision expert Bill Adaway, who was just about to set up a new, high-tech image-processing company. Together, we fought BTG and after much argument persuaded them to issue a reasonably priced license.

This also helped Bill raise venture capital for his company. He and his colleagues redesigned the WISARD using modern microchip technology, and the first commercial WISARD was sold to the Home Office for fingerprint recognition in 1984. WISARD was not a huge commercial success, but established the fact that digital neural networks were a usable tool. Variants of it crept into several systems built in the computer industry and government research establishments. WISARD techniques were used in crowd assessment machines for underground platforms, banknote-counting machines used the world over, railway-junction monitoring systems, and military-vehicle recognition devices. The first tentative experiments with Sophia at the University of Kent sixteen years previously had now paid off. Or had they?

A Change of Direction?

I could not put my finger on the reason, but I started feeling an anticlimactic depression about the seeming success of WISARD. It had something to do with the fact that the dream of studying systems with effective inner representations of the world had receded.

WISARD had no inner representation; it was just an efficient but massively dumb image-labeling system. It was as if *real* neural brains, with their awesome powers of providing the inner world of our own selves, were saying, "There. We told you so! Try to imitate us and you end up with gadgets that are not like us at all!" The thought was daunting of going through the grind of proving yet another set of neural principles as different from WISARD as WISARD was different from conventional computing. Even less appealing was the thought of designing and building yet another machine in a funding environment that, despite WISARD, had become hostile to unconventional techniques. Government was developing macho attitudes toward research in computing. The Alvey program was under pressure to prove its importance to industry. Conventional rule-based programming now represented an enormously heavy investment in what, from my perspective, were rather obvious and limited computing techniques.

The decisive event, which provided a choice for my future, was an invitation in 1984 to Imperial College in London to give a talk to electrical engineering researchers (on the WISARD, of course). Over lunch, the then head of the department, Bruce Sayers, asked whether I would be interested in a vacant Chair funded by a private endowment and the Department of Trade and Industry. The task was to set up a unit at the college that would research ways of transferring information technology into the running of businesses so as to make them more effective. Bruce Sayers thought that my experience in technology transfer with the WISARD would be appropriate.

This seemed an interesting challenge. Within a few days I had said that I would be interested. I was interviewed and offered the position. I accepted. I was to be the inaugural Kobler Professor for the Management of Information Technology. The unit was named after Freddy Kobler who, having achieved financial success in the hotel industry in the United Kingdom, wanted to help a stumbling U.K. economy. The acceptance of this position meant that consciousness in machines would have to wait.

10

Starting the Week with Consciousness

It would not be too strong to speak of too many of today's scientists having something of an apostolic mission. They want to explain, at least, the wonders of their world. . . . Scientists began to appear on Start the Week *in greater and greater numbers.*

—Melvyn Bragg, *On Giants' Shoulders*[1]

With some trepidation, I have used the names of real protagonists of the consciousness debate in this chapter. I have tried to express their views and they, kindly, let me have some observations on the way I had done this. I apologize to them if some inaccuracies still exist and urge the reader to turn to quoted references to appreciate what my contributors really think.

—Igor Aleksander

―――――――

Broadcasting House

Many are not aware of the back entrance in Hallam Street of the grand edifice that is the BBC's Broadcasting House. But this is the way in to the studios in which programs such as *Start the Week* are produced. I was there to do something else, but was told that there would be a delay. Would I mind sitting down and waiting? It could be as long as half an hour. Ho hum . . . It brought back a memory of many vivid discussions that had taken place on that program in the past. It was no longer done in the same way. But, strangely, when the young researcher came back, she said, "You can come in now. Melvyn and the others are in the studio already."

Starting the Millennium

"Are you all comfortable?" asked Melvyn Bragg. "After the news, we'll start." There was a vague rumbling of agreement around the large, baize-covered table bedecked with microphones covered in colorful plastic shields. The newsreader summarized the latest scandal and reported yet another victim of the Year 2000 problem: Southern Railways claimed that they were sold the wrong kind of computer, but luckily it would mark as "on time" all trains that were up to an hour late, so don't bother trying to obtain compensation . . .

BRAGG: Good morning and welcome to the first *Start the Week* of the millennium. A "Start the Millennium" indeed. The topic before us is probably the greatest puzzle of the last millennium, which shows no sign of abating in this one: consciousness, is it safe in the hands of scientists? We have brought together many of those who have written on the topic and pronounced on it, sometimes vociferously, in the media.

Susan Greenfield[2] is a professor of pharmacology at Oxford and is giving a series of lectures at the Royal Institution on "What Happens to Consciousness When We Go Bungee-Jumping?" Roger Penrose[3] is Rouse Ball Professor of Mathematics at the University of Oxford, and has just published a new book, *Non-Computation: An Essential Science*. Steven Rose[4] is Professor of Biology at the Open University. His lecture for the Royal Society this week is entitled "Filing Cabinets Cannot be Conscious." Margaret Boden is a psychologist, a philosopher, and a prolific author who specializes in explaining and analyzing the philosophy of scientists in the Artificial Intelligence and Artificial Life domains. Her latest book is called *The Neural Coincidence*. Aaron Sloman, a philosopher, is also a professor of Artificial Intelligence and Cognitive Science at Birmingham University and has just published *Ethics for Conscious Computers*. And Igor Aleksander is Professor of Neural Engineering at Imperial College, whose book *How to Build a Mind* will be published later this year.

But that is just the British contingent. From the United States we have imported Francis Crick, Nobel Laureate, who with Christof Koch has just published the book *Astonishingly Conscious Neurons*. Daniel Dennett is a philosopher at Tufts University in Boston and has a TV series, "The Myth of the Cartesian Theater," gracing our British screens at the moment. And Steven Pinker is a psychologist at MIT whose recent massive one-thousand-page book, *Consciousness for the Masses*, has broken all sales records.

We have an hour, so I shall begin by bringing you in one at a time. Then we shall see how things develop. Francis Crick, you have been scathing about philosophers and their achievements. Where do you stand at the moment?

CRICK: It may well be that the philosophers got there first in being fascinated by what they called "soul" and then "consciousness." But they did so for the nature of matter, the movement of stellar bodies, and the growth of plants. Nonetheless, it is the physicist, the cosmologist, and the biologist who have discovered the laws that explain these phenomena and enable us to control our existence among the elements. Sadly, the philosophers' record over the last two thousand years has been so poor that I do not have much hope that they will make a major contribution to solving the problem of consciousness. Philosophers are good at asking interesting questions, some of which may point in the right direction, but history has shown that they have no technique for providing really satisfactory answers to them. Christof Koch's next book will try to outline the problem in scientific terms, but we are still far from glimpsing the answers, let alone providing the correct ones.

BRAGG: The poor record of philosophers? Margaret Boden, you straddle the philosophy-science divide. Do philosophers need to be educated?

BODEN: Philosophy is alive and well and, may I say it, robust enough to withstand these attacks. This does not mean that what scientists do is pointless—of course they discover the laws of physics, chemistry, and neurophysiology, but consciousness is much harder to explain. They cannot explain everything. You would not go to a scientist for an explanation of the causes of poverty in India or why the First World War started . . . Consciousness is essentially a construct in the study of humanity. What Francis and his colleagues do is merely to study the essentials that make consciousness possible. A well-working brain is undoubtedly needed in order for someone to be an intelligent, conscious human being.

So neurophysiologists may indeed be able to tell us what constitutes a well-working brain and what happens when there are deficits. When they note that blood flows in a particular bit of brain when the patient is conscious of something specific, this is merely a measure of correlation and not an explanation of how the subject feels anything at all. Measuring the flow of petrol in a particular part of a car does not explain how a car works. But in the case of a car, mechanical engineering exists to give us a full explanation. Indeed in good old-fashioned Artificial Intelligence, logic and programming exist to define an intelligent act, such as playing chess. This is not based on the engineering of the microchips in the computer. But to explain consciousness, the equivalent of logic and computation does not exist. It will be many years—and perhaps never—before a totally new and currently unimaginable science is developed to explain consciousness.

BRAGG: Daniel Dennett, you seemed to be getting agitated while Margaret was speaking. Of course, you have written a book called *Consciousness Explained*. So, have you cracked it?

DENNETT: It's not that difficult, Melvyn. Make no mistake, I am a philosopher. And it is precisely by embracing some models from computation that I as a philosopher find a language that expresses what consciousness is. The thought of sitting around and waiting for someone to invent a new science to bridge some strange gap is just good old-fashioned dualism! It is precisely the mistake that Descartes made, and many others make, in discussing consciousness. The idea that consciousness is like a movie that goes on in our heads (what I call Cartesian Theater) and that the owner of that head is the sole member of the audience, has the obvious problem of infinite regress. What is the consciousness with which the observer watches the movie? There is no Cartesian Theater and I am not the first to say this—Wittgenstein said it more forcefully than anyone else.

The brain is a very fine and evolved instrument, made up of many specialist parts. Think of the metaphor of a newspaper office that is producing a newspaper on a continuous basis, with editors revising and editing stories as they come in. Similarly, virtual computational agents generated by our brains edit the newspaper of consciousness. Consciousness is just a state of part of this computing process that is analogous to the current state of the newspaper. But this state need not be "read"; it is the current state of part of the brain. But I have said that all these editors and the newspaper are "virtual." They form what computer people call a multi-agent system. I can press a button on my computer, and lo and behold a calculator appears on the screen: this is a single virtual agent. With my mouse I can press its buttons and get a result just like on the calculator in my pocket. My model of consciousness is a multi-agent virtual machine running on a neural substrate, forged by evolution to revise continually the drafts of a story as sensory experience comes in. There is no gap, there is no special internal, unexplainable entity such as a "Quale." There is no need to find a science that explains something that is a figment of mistaken philosophers' logic.

BRAGG: I'm not sure that I understand all that. Aaron Sloman, you are both a philosopher and an artificial intelligence expert. Can you unravel this for us a bit?

SLOMAN: I actually find that Daniel's "explanation" is not an explanation. It is, rather, a statement of intent or a framework—a language for an explanation. It is a structure within which, with a lot of hard work, you might fashion an explanation. To say that a car is a vehicle driven by a petrol-combustion engine does not tell us how a car works; it only points to some other science (the design and operation of internal combustion engines) within which it is possible to explain what makes a car go. Virtual agents are just metaphors that refer to certain styles of programming; they are expressions of something understood and worked through by a programmer. A virtual agent is just a free-standing chunk of program with a well-defined behavior.

But this working-through still needs to be done—it is the research that I do. In my work, I am trying, as far as possible, to define and refine the requirements for programs that encompass what is known about things such as attention, recognition, and even emotions such as "love." This leads to a system made up of many interacting programs, which as a whole might have some of the characteristics of the agglomeration of things we call "consciousness." The notion of editors and a newspaper as a model of consciousness is an amusing metaphor, but does not help me in my work. When I finish what I am trying to do, it may well be the case that we shall have a computer that has a sufficiently strongly expressed sense of self for its friends, teachers, pupils, employers, and coworkers to believe that it has some form of consciousness. We may even have to think carefully of what rights it can and should demand.

BRAGG: Roger Penrose, I would expect you to disagree.

PENROSE: Indeed, I have great reservations about any form of explanation that suggests that the brain can be likened to a computer or that a computer can emulate the way that the brain provides us with our consciousness. One of the many fascinating characteristics of our consciousness is what we might call "insight." This comes from our ability to face, in our minds, several alternatives at once, and to jump to a suitable thought in a way that would be impossible for a computer. For example, when studying geometry, the bright student will often ask, "How did Euclid know which steps need to be taken to prove a theorem?" This question is central to what Gödel has said about proofs of theorems in general. He refers to a formal system, such as Euclidean geometry, and shows that to prove all its theorems the human has to step outside the formal system and have insight that cannot be obtained from within the system. Now, Turing has shown that a computer can only do less than or, at best, as much as can be done from within a formal system created by a programmer. So, I come to the conclusion that any science that claims to explain consciousness will have to go beyond what can be computed, because it will have to combine being within the formal system and being outside it at the same time.

There is only one corner of physics in which something like this can be computed and it is in the area of quantum physics. Here, it is commonplace to think of a complex system as being in a variety of states until a measurement is made. The neural state of the brain, in common with the state of a computer, does not exhibit this property. I therefore find it hard to believe that explanations of consciousness that are based on only the functioning of neurons in the brain hold the answer. They are constrained by the same laws as computers. There are, however, structures in nerve cells within which there is a hope of finding such quantum effects. These are called "microtubules." Without going further, I have to say that even if microtubules have the correct quantum characteristics of being able to enter one of several potential states, the process cannot be random. Some simply say that the freedom of will comes from random noise among the neurons. Will is free but not random. The scientific principles for this are at present unknown.

Consciousness is just too important to believe that it is something accidentally conjured up by computation in our brains.

BRAGG: Both Margaret and Roger then believe that we do not yet have the tools to explain consciousness. What worries me is that all the effort that is being exerted by neurobiologists and neural modelers at the moment may prove to be a waste of time. Igor Aleksander, will your work become redundant?

ALEKSANDER: Not in the next few days, I hope. At the end of it all, the methods we all use for gaining insights into consciousness are personal and based on our individual skills. I find that what neurobiologists discover about the way in which physical, unashamedly neural and not microtubular, events in the brain relate to the sensation reported by the subject is the sanest avenue toward gaining usable insights into how those very sensations are generated. It provides invaluable data both to guide and verify our computer simulations.

The computational nature of theories or simulations of these processes is not a constraining factor; indeed it has the power to explain the nature of "insight" that Roger is looking for. It predicts the occurrence of certain sensations and formulates the conditions under which they arise. It is quite possible for a neural network to be in an overall state that represents several solutions to a problem, but then to jump to the appropriate way forward. Roger's attack on the computational limitations of Turing machines is quite correct but misplaced: used as a simulator, a computer can represent both a formal system and the way it can find solutions, which cannot be proved within that system. That is, it allows us to study systems, such as complex neural networks, that do "jump to conclusions." The use of the word "coincidence" or "correlation" between neural behavior and sensation used by Margaret creates an unnecessary gap between the two. The theories that link them have been with us for some time, as I explain in the last chapter of the book I am writing.

BRAGG: We shall have to hold our breath! Steven Pinker, you were looking anxious when Roger was speaking.

PINKER: Yes, I think that Igor was being too kind to Roger. As I have explained in my books, his ideas are not valid. He confuses the behavior of an idealized mathematician with a real, live and conscious one who may be influenced by analogy, personal preference, and experience way outside the theorems he is trying to prove. So, insight comes very much from experience and does not suffer from the Gîdelian limitations on which Roger bases his argument. Also, there is no hint of how consciousness might emerge from quantum mechanics.

But I don't agree with Igor either. He falls into the trap that all neuroscientists inhabit: he confuses explaining the way in which the brain allows access to experience with explaining "sentience," the "I" in consciousness. Once all the neural-theoretical predictions have been worked out, will sentience no longer be a puzzle? The heck it will not. It will remain untouched. The major unanswered questions will not vanish. If Igor's simulation gets so good that it predicts what people feel when you tweak some of their neurons, will his virtual machine be conscious? Could your experience of red be the same as mine of green? Could there be zombies—could an artificial model of me, accurate in every detail and programmed to act like me, exist without feeling or seeing anything? What is it like to be a bat? If I replace your neurons one by one by exact copies, but have them made in silicon, at what point do you become an automaton, a thing without consciousness?

I just can't answer these questions even if Igor gives me a full predictive theory of what causes representations in my head. It just may be that we were built in a way where, despite our advancing science, these remain unanswerable questions. And it may be a good thing too: this inability may be part of the characteristics of mind that go with enjoying jokes, enthusing about a new performance of the Prokofiev Violin Concerto, or savoring some wine. It could be the characteristic that makes mind worth having. There is a big difference between how the mind works, which is an evolved process with strong computational characteristics, and explaining how it appears to us when it is in full activity.

BRAGG: Steve Rose, you have displayed just a tad of antagonism to Steve Pinker's views in your reviews of his books, so, what do you think?

ROSE: While I applaud Steve's stance that mechanistic explanations still leave many questions unanswered, I shudder when he uses the word "evolved." This comes back to a kind of "Swiss Army knife" view of how the mind works: a computational tool for everything to go with a gene for everything. This is genetic determinism gone wild. In fact, the formation of what we call "the mind" is the result of an exquisite interplay between genes and the superb capacity of the brain mechanisms to change and develop during our lifetimes. To turn this into a computational model is a deeply flawed idea.

The way that changes in the brain happen in a purposive way needs to be understood by knowing how evolutionary processes are influenced by emotion, societal issues, and meanings imposed by these. This does not need to be modeled in a foreign medium such as computation, which only results in a dehumanized view of ourselves. In the last analysis, to understand the brain we must study the brain. Igor's machine will never be "conscious" in any meaningful way; Pinker's mind is not a mechanistic product of ontogenesis; and Daniel Dennett would not be the elegant author he is were he to rely only on some evolved multi-agent newspaper-producing machine.

But let me finish by attacking my favorite target: the way in which neuroscience assumes the character of a power tool. There is a danger that some of its more reductionist aspects have the potential of adjusting our mental traits to suit the world. There is an increasing confidence within those who are looking at genes to explain through them stress, crime, anxiety, alcohol dependency, sexual orientation, and even poverty. The danger in this assumption is that, through an acceptance of these models, minds can be controlled, consciousnesses adjusted, and people made to submit, through chemical manipulation, to the waywardness of some political obduracy.

BRAGG: Susan Greenfield, you are a pharmacologist, so this could not be a more appropriate point at which to bring you in.

GREENFIELD: Thank you. Yes, how fascinating. All this supports a point

I often make. Your guests all have their own ideas about how mind emerges from brain. This proves that no one has an answer that is unequivocally acceptable. So we are not there yet. We may, indeed, be a long way from anything like an accepted understanding of consciousness. The essence of science is objectivity. A theory of consciousness must embrace subjectivity; this is why the classical scientific establishment is prepared to zap anyone who claims to be interested in the subject. But the answer must lie in the neurons. Not Igor's artificial neural nets—messing about with computers gets you nowhere.

I agree with Steve: to discover consciousness, you need to study the brain in all its squishy, chemical glory. There is an epicenter where sensation comes in. This recruits assemblies of neurons. We feel things in sequence, so consciousness is spatially multiple and temporally unitary. There is a continuum in consciousness from the minimal to the profound. A young child is conscious but not in the same sophisticated way as George Bernard Shaw, or, toward the other extreme, a rat. A human adult's consciousness changes from morning to evening. It is different at a rave or while having sex. Neuronal assemblies could be small, leading to an absorbing obsession with sensory input— possibly what is happening in schizophrenia. But they could be large, leading to distant, blurred views of the world. So I conclude that there is no magic. Much insight will be gained when one can actually measure the size and behavior of active neuronal assemblies and relate them to the sensation felt by the volunteer. I predict that, with the advance of time- and space-resolution in brain-imaging techniques, my models will be confirmed and give us a purchase on a true science of consciousness.

BRAGG: Well, on that positive and upbeat note, let me open the discussion. We do not have much time left so may I ask you to add to the discussion, bearing the listener in mind. From where I am sitting I get a feeling of a major divide between those who think that science has a grip on consciousness and those who feel that the grip can at best be partial or, at worst, impossible. I would appreciate it if you could tell me how this divide might be narrowed in the future or whether it is inherent in the concept, a product of the very difference in our personalities.

PENROSE: I am optimistic about the future. The sterility of current approaches drives us to seek new insights. For this reason, those offering explanations of consciousness now should not be afraid to face the limitations of what they are saying.

BODEN: I would say that in this group there is much agreement that science is inadequate, while philosophy is useful in keeping some real questions helpfully alive.

CRICK: That's just nonsense. Science is quite capable of keeping the real questions alive and, eventually, solving them, though a little help from the philosophers might be welcomed. What is mainly needed is less talk and more relevant experiments and, even more important, new and better experimental methods. We shall also need new ideas, but I rather doubt that they will be as radical as, for example, Penrose's ideas.

GREENFIELD: There's no big equation that zaps the problem. Also the current fad to do science by button-pushing and computers is something that we shall have to grow out of. It simply creates a wall of former Berlin proportions between the reality of needing to understand the biochemical basis of qualia and some vague modeling that simply restates the problem. A study of consciousness is anathema for the scientific establishment, and so those of us who are doing it seriously get confused with the modelers who do nothing.

SLOMAN: Now that's an admission of not understanding the process of modeling if ever I heard one. How can we argue that the scientific establishment does not understand us when we sling mud at each other. The more the so-called "natural" scientists grasp computer modeling as one of the many exceedingly powerful tools that are available to gain an understanding of the great questions, the sooner will the questions start gathering answers.

Computer modeling is no different from the modeling that good physicists and chemists have done for centuries.

ROSE: I don't like computers either. They distract us from the point that consciousness is a human question asked of living objects.

DENNETT: That could just be envy. Yes, many questions remain unanswered, but the computer scientist and the mathematician have probably made more sense of complex systems such as the brain than any biologist or philosopher I know.

PINKER: Yes but the computer hacker who ignores the facts of life—in language for example—will produce vacuous models. Those of us who straddle the nature-computation divide are well-placed to make progress and be sensitive to what still needs to be said.

BRAGG: I see no more hands, just worried faces. Have we concluded that there is no consensus, therefore no paradigm is in sight? Igor Aleksander, you have gone remarkably quiet. It's your turn.

I froze. My head was spinning. Nine pairs of eyes were on me. Nobody seemed keen to hear about the emergent properties of complex systems, how consciousness might be one such property of the brain, or how understanding machines might be a way to get to grips with this. I knew that anything I said would merely unify the others in condemning the word "emergent." In a hoarse voice I said "Not now . . . Read the last chapter . . ."

Escape

"It's your turn now, Professor Aleksander . . ."

Who is this? Where am I? Ah yes, the back of Broadcasting House. This earnest young woman was the person who said that there was going to be a delay. How long had I been asleep? "We're ready for you," she went on. "Professor Reading of Warwick has just completed recording a fascinating discourse on how implanting chips in our brains will equip us to fight the wars against conscious robots—like the ones you are making for example. So what we want from you is just a sound bite on when the first conscious robot will roll off the production lines. Can you tell me now what your sound bite is?"

"Er . . . er . . . sound   bite? . . . Wars? . . . Conscious robots?" I stammered. I produced my sound bite: "Could someone call me a taxi, it's time I went home."

MAGNUS in South Kensington and Pasadena

MAGNUS "lives" in a virtual environment that simulates the real world as closely as possible. The environment exerts its own demands, and this is what provides stimulus, or motivation, without which there would be no activity.

—Jasia Reichardt, in *Frankenstein, Creation and Monstrosity*[1]

Imperial College: A Quarter of a Century Late

My first day at Imperial College seemed like the fulfillment of a long-standing aim. After all, my purpose in coming to England in 1958 was to do research at this college. Driving through Hyde Park on that first morning twenty-six years later, I actually found the slow traffic a boon. The early sun was seeping through the mist, giving the odd horse and rider trotting past the traffic an incongruous, surreal aura. It gave me time to reflect on how to manage my research. In the previous months, since knowing of my appointment, I had put in place a few projects that would enable me to look at the management of information technology as a series of important questions.

The central one was what differentiates a firm that has done better by using computers from one that has done worse (of which there were many). Although obvious, the answer (prompted by our guru from the United States, Paul Strassman of the Xerox Corporation) lay in applying machines to improve the effectiveness of the firm, that is, improving the quality of whatever the firm was doing. Those who used machines to reduce costs (firing people and reducing services to suit the computer) were doomed to failure.

While these principles had little to do with technology or, indeed, cognitive science, neural systems were becoming increasingly important in the general world of computer science. It thus became possible for me to maintain research in this area as a facet of the management of information technology.

The Connectionist Fashion

The first sign that American scientists were beginning to renew their interest in neural networks came with the publication of two seminal papers by John Hopfield, one in 1982 and the other in 1984.[2] They clearly referred to systems with feedback and internal states and so, bearing in mind that my entire experience pointed to this as being the major issue in neural networks, it made me prick up my ears. Hopfield provided an elegant analysis of such systems, which likened the state of a feedback net to a ball on a smooth sheet with circular dips in it. These dips are the learned, stable (i.e., unchanging in time) states of the system—a most helpful analogy.

Whether it was John Hopfield's influence or not, it suddenly became fashionable (and, indeed, forcefully so) for some U.S. workers to hold up neural methods as alternatives to knowledge-based systems, because the latter had proved to be problematic in difficult pattern-recognition areas and natural language processing. The banner of this revival was a cure to the disease uncovered by Minsky and Papert fifteen or so years earlier: the limitations of the so-called "single layer perceptron" and the demolition job they did on Frank Rosenblatt's ideas (see chapter 7). The cure lay in using more than one layer: two, in fact, in addition to the input layer. This middle layer (known as the "hidden layer") rearranges the information arriving at the input so as to make tractable problems normally intractable for a single output layer.

While it has always been known that a hidden layer could perform this magic, there seemed to be no obvious way of making it do this as part of a learning and training procedure. Several people (for example, Geoff Hinton at Carnegie Mellon, and Paul Werbos of NASA) hit upon an idea for solving this problem. The technique was given the horrid name of "error back-propagation." As the name implies, it was a way of adjusting the functions of the neurons in the hidden layer by causing errors at the output layer to propagate backwards, providing information as to how much the middle needed to change. That's it—no more needs to be said.

It so happened that Geoff Hinton, an Englishman who had gone to the United States, spent a short sabbatical in my group at Imperial College. It was short because Geoff became disenchanted with the poor level of e-mail service that Imperial could provide in 1985. More interesting than his disenchantment was the fact that he was developing an improved form of Hopfield net called the Boltzmann machine. The Hopfield net had a characteristic that could cause it not to find a trained state, because, on the way down to the bottom of a dip, it might find a local dip where it would get stuck. Mathematicians call this the "false minimum" problem. Hinton was working on a system in which he would introduce a reducing amount of electronic disturbance ("noise" in the language of electronics). This would effectively shake the ball out of the false dip into the real one.

All of this merely served to increase my desire to get back into working with dynamic neural nets. Hinton was most critical of my digital approach, largely because much of what was happening in error back-propagation and Hopfield/Boltzmann nets, achieved a certain mathematical elegance through its being a bit like the dips and hills of a smooth physical system. Here the gentle slopes of continuous physical functions contrast with the dirty abruptness of digital systems. But, for me, the fact that a digital net with feedback behaved in much the same way as a Hopfield net, but could not be explained by Hopfield analysis, was a stimulant to curiosity. It meant that there was a need to look at mathematical laws that were more general than those used in the physics of nondigital systems. It seemed most unlikely that energy equations could be written to encompass the complex architectures of the brain. There is not much likelihood of "hidden layers" in the brain either. So, despite the revival, young researchers in the United States seemed to be beginning to plow furrows based on the "multilayer perceptron" and dynamic nets that relied on the sheet-with-dips idea. But that would divert the effort from studying what the brain may be doing.

On the Fringe Again

In 1986, Geoff Hinton contributed his ideas to a pair of books edited by cognitive scientists David Rumelhart and Jay McClelland that went under the title of Parallel Distributed Processing (PDP).[3] The word *connectionist* became a fashionable way of describing neural systems, and ways of adjusting connection weights between neurons became seen as one of the foci of inquiry in the field. The PDP books became the bibles of a rapidly growing community of young researchers captivated by the refreshing novelty of doing computation with continuous and parallel systems as opposed to the digital style of the serial computer. Conferences such as the 1987 International Conference on Neural Networks and the 1988 International Joint Conference on Neural Networks in San Diego were attracting a huge number of delegates.

The organizers of such conferences also began to discover that there were some old hands in the field: Bernie Widrow of Stanford, who invented a net called the Adaline in the 1960s; Stephen Grossberg of Boston University; James Anderson of Brown University; and Walter Freeman of Berkeley, who had been developing a wide variety of dynamic neural models of neurobiological systems in the 1970s. The discovery of this earlier work led to relationships among workers that were not always harmonious. The only European who was known to the emerging U.S. connectionists was the Finnish pioneer of associative neural systems, Teuvo Kohonen. He was invited to the 1988 San Diego conference, where he spoke of the work of European workers such as myself, John Taylor of King's College, London, and Eduardo Caianiello, a doyen of the field from Salerno in Italy. In Japan, too, American researchers discovered the mathematically superb work of Shun Ichi Amari of Tokyo University.

But for me, as the scientific world was beginning to turn its head toward neural networks again, because of my interest in digital and cognitive neural systems I was once more outside the mainstream of the new neural-network fashion. The mainstream was developing in the world of mathematics as used in physics. I felt that this was a narrowing and stultifying approach that focused on pattern-recognition applications or very simple dynamic systems, when the real excitement lay in trying to unravel the intricate architecture of the brain, and its ability—well, yes—to think and be conscious.

Personally I found this felt very much as things had done earlier when I was advocating neural networks to computing scientists hell-bent on rule-based AI systems. Now I was advocating a study of architectures of systems with inner states that, in a digital world, represent sensory experience. And I was advocating it to people hell-bent on improving error back-propagation systems in a world of continuous mathematics. Although the PDP books had chapters on networks that performed cognitive functions, they looked suspiciously like neural implementations of ideas that were spawned during the AI rule-based era.

Back into Engineering

It was a Friday in the spring of 1988, and I had just given a paper at a computer vision conference in Cambridge. Someone said, "There's an urgent call for you from Imperial College." It was Sir Eric Ash, the then rector of the college: "I would like you to be the next head of the Electrical Engineering Department," he said.

"Can I come and see you on Monday so that we can talk about

it?" I said (playing for time, so that I could think and discuss it with Helen).

"No," he said. "I want you to phone me this afternoon with your answer. After all, you have done this kind of thing before at Brunel."

I went for a long walk along the banks of the Cam. The responsibility was enormous but the offer could not be more attractive. One idea that gave me a specific buzz was the thought of being head of the department where Colin Cherry had done his work—the man who made me come to Britain in the first place. This department was one of the best in the country and one that had spawned many engineers who were applying their skills in the life sciences as a result of the influence of Colin Cherry, Eric Laithwaite, and Dennis Gabor. But a little voice at the back of my mind was asking whether this would put an end to my rising ambition to study neural nets with mindlike properties.

"Not in the least," said Eric Ash when I next spoke to him. "Most heads of Imperial departments are research stars, so I would support your efforts to set up a neural laboratory." I agreed to take up the post. It turned out later that my Chair would be named the Gabor Chair in recognition of the work of Nobel Laureate Dennis Gabor, who had been one of the exceptional researchers of that department. So I became the Gabor Professor of Neural Systems Engineering and head of the Electrical Engineering Department, a post I was to hold for nine years. The Kobler mantle was to be ably taken up by Bruce Sayers, when he came to the end of his stint as head of the Department of Computing, and by Catherine Griffiths, a bright researcher with an education in the Classics.

WISARD and a Mental Image

After a year or so of getting to grips with Resources and Budget Committees, Course Development Committees, College Heads' meetings, the Annual Financial Plan, and the needs of colleagues and students, the odd chink of time began to appear for getting back to the design of neural systems. With Adrian Redgers, a bright physicist whom I had known since he was a child, we got a grant to buy a commercial WISARD. Within this we introduced feedback loops so that, rather than recognize patterns, it would be able to represent them and reconstruct them from cues coming in from its TV camera "eye." But before we could do this we had to solve a problem that exists in all neural systems with feedback, including the brain. How do these representations (mental images, we may wish to call them) get into the feedback loops of the system?

We thought of a very simple system, which had a binary eye of 8 × 8 (64) black/white picture points. This fed a neural net with at least 64 large neurons arranged in an 8 × 8 array. As we had known since the Sophia days of the late 1960s, the firing patterns of these neurons were transmitted back to the inputs in order to have any memory at all. So this is where a major part of our philosophy about inner states had to be developed, and it was simplicity itself. The inner states had to represent seen images. So if an 8 × 8 image had to be learned, it had not only to be present at the eye but also had to find its way to the terminals that teach the neurons to fire or not. We called this "iconic" learning. Adrian managed to twist the WISARD into doing this and demonstrated not only that this digital system had useful "dips," as in Hopfield nets, but also fell into these dips when "seeing" partial cues through its eye. The dips themselves formed the "mental images" that WISARD could use. This behavior was filmed for a Central Office of Information program as a way of unmasking a masked criminal just from a view of his eyes. The WISARD, instead of saying, "It is Fred (as opposed to Jack, Jill, or John)," as it did in the past, would now say two things: "I know this image," and, "This is what I think the man looks like." The recognition of the face could always be done in the old way.

So this may have been the very first time that an iconic learning system was made to work and produce a "mental image" for an artificial system, but at what a price! WISARD was a sledgehammer not designed to crack this particular nut. Putting aside any implications that this may or may not have had for saying how mental imagery arises in our heads, it was clear that if such phenomena were to be properly studied, a different way had to be found. Continuing to work with our colleagues at Brunel, Adrian and I began to formulate a new approach: a system which was built to create many modules capable of inner representation (automata) of sufficient generality to be able easily to study mental events such as imagery and its relation to language. It was thus that a Multi-Automata, General Neural Unified Structure, or MAGNUS, was born (even though, admittedly, the mnemonic was somewhat painfully contrived).

MAGNUS: A Tool for Brain Modeling

After some considerable to-ing and fro-ing with the research funding agency (EPSRC), we got a grant to construct this new machine. The EPSRC was now convinced about neural nets for pattern recognition, but was skeptical of our "biologically inspired" approach and only swayed by our argument that we might some day improve the performance of robots. But even before the money arrived, we realized that any thought of doing this in hardware was a stupid idea. Serial software operating on really fast laboratory computers had become so powerful that it was clearly the method to use; it would be less expensive and far more powerful than hardware. So we assembled a team of excellent software engineers to get the job done. They were Panos Ntourntoufis and William Penny at Brunel, with Adrian Redgers and Richard Evans at Imperial College. It was 1989, and it would take three years to develop this system.

The specification included the facility that a user could build not only a multi-automata neural structure but also the "virtual visual world" in which the neural organisms could "live." These are rather exaggerated ways of describing the fact that MAGNUS would be designed so as to receive as input an image seen through a "window" on a world that, in itself, was stored in the host computer—that is, a virtual world. It could also move this input around this world and learn to develop planning strategies for this kind of exploration.

The Mind of Yorick

While MAGNUS was being planned and designed, we could not resist tinkering with hardware. The problem with developing a major machine as a virtual software object is that whatever organism we generated it would fall prey to the "it's only a computer" criticism: it can only do what the programmer tells it. The concept of a virtual machine is hard to grasp: the host computer in MAGNUS would, to all intents and purposes, be like the neural net it emulates. The user would indeed be able to put together a neural system in much the way a child might construct a windmill with an Erector set. When the windmill whirls in the wind according to the laws of aerodynamics, it transcends its Erector-set character. So it is with a virtual neural net; it behaves according to the laws of emergent neural dynamics and transcends the fact that it is hosted by a dumb computer.

But to prove the point that the computer is an irrelevant and transparent tool in the affair, we decided to build another neural system with a visible "mental image" display on an array of light-emitting diodes (such as those used nowadays on indicator boards on underground stations). There would not be a computer in sight. The system was designed and built by Jim Lucy, a research student who, tragically, died in an accident just after the project was completed. Jim had chosen a plastic skull into which he fitted his creation. This had photocell eyes and showed off, once the top of the skull had been removed, a glowing image of a sunny day or a night scene, depending on which of two related images it was "observing."

Exhibits such as this attract television film crews. In this case, a team from the British TV show *Equinox* was visiting the laboratory to film the WISARD doing its reconstructing of masked faces. But, seeing the skull, they much preferred it and dubbed it "Yorick" in the program.

This was the occasion on which, while I was being interviewed to explain these inner images, the show's host suggested that, because Yorick could visualize what it was seeing, it might be conscious. I protested strenuously on camera: "Consciousness is for living creatures, not artificial objects." My mind was racing wildly and I continued: "I suppose . . . that if an artificial object could somehow become aware of its environment, one could say it was 'conscious' in a highly artificial way." This was the moment when the seemingly incongruous idea of an artificial consciousness came into being. Did the concept make sense? Would it elucidate real consciousness? These questions were to remain with me for a long time.

Yorick eventually became exhibited in the 1992 Faraday Lecture arranged by the Institution of Electrical Engineers (in which it was called "Igor"), and then, in 1996 it became an exhibit as an example of contemporary neural network research in the Science Museum. Jim Lucy continues to be sadly missed in my laboratory.

Consciousness: A Fashionable Topic

The reason that the program's host had asked whether my artificial neural nets were conscious was because Roger Penrose's book *The Emperor's New Mind* had recently been published.[4] This made the strong point that consciousness was something that was beyond the reach of computation—or, indeed, any known science. This started a philosophical and scientific controversy that still resonates at the time of writing (autumn 1999) and is likely to do so for some time to come. Other books followed: Daniel Dennett's *Consciousness Explained* in 1991,[5] and Francis Crick's *The Astonishing Hypothesis* in 1994.[6] The latter two disagreed with Penrose in different ways, Dennett arguing that computational metaphors were appropriate, and Crick seeing it as a hard-nosed neurophysiological problem. All I knew was that a growing interest in artificial consciousness was like jumping into a very deep and muddy pool with an underdeveloped aptitude for swimming. Many advised me against it, some suggested that it would ruin my scientific credibility, and some shrugged their shoulders saying, "He's just getting old. He can't hack the hard stuff any more!"

But the more I was advised against it, the more I became convinced that, armed with an understanding of the emerging engineering properties of complex cellular systems, I could contribute something to the debate. Interestingly, all of the above exponents agreed that consciousness could be explained in some material way. But none of them considered that the most direct way of doing this might be to ask what distinguishes a neural structure that generates consciousness from one that does not, and that this problem could be approached through artificial neural networks. I was sure that I had a new perspective to add to the burgeoning debate on consciousness.

The Colin Cherry Lecture

Robert Spence was—and is—one of the professors in my new home in the Electrical Engineering Department. He had been one of Colin Cherry's students and was busy doing research in human-machine interaction. He is making great contributions to the improvement of the way data are presented on screens to engineers who are engaged in the design of complex systems. To do this, in the Cherry tradition, he started by making models of what is known of human perception and the cognition that this involves, which led him to develop user-adapted displays. He and Bruce Sayers (also a former research fellow of Cherry's) decided to found an annual lecture in Cherry's memory: the Colin Cherry Memorial Lecture.

In 1992 they asked me to deliver this lecture. I was delighted to accept. I gave it the purposely ambiguous title of "Imagining Machines" and, in my opening slide, suggested that consciousness was a proper subject for study, particularly under the umbrella of artificial neural networks. Margaret Boden, the philosopher from Sussex University, was in the audience, and was heard to whisper on the way out: "Interesting, but he was nowhere near even understanding what consciousness *is*!" Clearly, I had joined the club—a philosopher had disagreed with me. The consciousness club is one in which people make their name when others disagree with them.

The MAGNUS Completed

The researchers working on the MAGNUS began to demonstrate it working in early 1992. It was in June of that year that the system was exhibited at a soirée at the Royal Society—exactly ten years after the WISARD had been exposed to similar scrutiny. The salient advance with this system was that it had an inner state with which it could represent a visual world in some detail. The power of the system began to depend on the power of the host computer. So, using some of the most powerful laboratory computers available at the time, we were able to work with an inner state of about 50,000 picture points (just over 200 × 200)—a pleasing advance over the 64 picture points available to the WISARD with feedback.

The early experiments with the system demonstrated inner ("mental") exploration. In the first of these the system was shown a set of objects placed in a row (cone, sphere, box). Then, while an object was being shown at the input and caused to make the inner neurons fire (in what was called the "iconic" way earlier in this book), the name was also added through a second input. The upshot of all this was that "with its eyes shut," given the name of an object, MAGNUS would visibly (recalling that its "thoughts" were displayed on a screen) imagine the object. But more than this, if given the name of another object, the thoughts would show the appropriate trajectory in space. That is, were there objects between the first and the second shape it would imagine them. While this was predictable, it was gratifying that it actually happened. Many other similar successful experiments convinced me that various effects involving mental representation were tiny pieces of the jigsaw that is called consciousness. This led me to begin writing *Impossible Minds*, which was published in 1996.[7] In this I could explain these fragments of insight in a relatively relaxed, nontechnical way. For completeness I summarize these arguments below.

Impossible Minds

As in this book, the starting point is that, inescapably, anything that we can think of, imagine, or plan—that is, the whole of our conscious existence—is the product of the firing of immensely complex assemblies of neurons. This, as anyone who has read Crick's *Astonishing Hypothesis* will realize, is a restatement of the hypothesis itself. The key question then becomes whether the mechanisms that create these patterns can be studied in an artificial domain such as MAGNUS. I argued positively, since to argue negatively would mean that some other, unknown forces were involved in generating these patterns. Another way of viewing this decision is to say, "let's see how far we can go with the analytical knowledge that we have, and only if this gets us nowhere will we agree with Penrose's contention that science currently does not offer the wherewithal to understand consciousness."

The scientific methodology I felt to be appropriate for an analysis in the artificial domain is automata theory—that is, the science of the internal state. This is concerned with calculating how an input into a machine made of known components causes an inner state to change. It also has an interesting mode of graphical representation whereby a state is drawn as a circle on a piece of paper and a state change due to an input as an arrow between states. The diagram of all possible transitions between states is what automata theoreticians call the "state structure" of machines with an inner state. While it seems obvious to say that mind is the state structure of part of the brain, this is also a pretty trivial thing to say because the number of states is so immeasurably huge, and the neural components that give rise to them are equally intractable. So the usefulness of automata theory lies in its ability to express specific aspects of consciousness in terms of the characteristics of state structures.

ι early consequence of this approach is that it may be possible ιο αistinguish three essential functional parts of the overall neural structure of the nervous system. These three types of neurons—which need not be in spatially distinct areas—comprise, first, those that maintain patterns of firing responsible for the sensation of a coherent world, and the imagining of such a world even if it is not being sensed. (It now seems necessary to leave open the possibility that a further physical separation between neurons for the perceptual and imaginatory elements of consciousness would be useful.) A second group of neurons adds inner events to those stimulated from the outside; a sense of sequence and timing is typical of the action of these neurons. The third set of neurons relates to control functions in the maintenance of the system, and their firing neither produces direct sensation nor is additional to the action of the sensation-generating neurons; in fact their activity does not enter consciousness at all but is still important because it controls functions such as breathing, heartbeat, and other physiological needs.

The activities of the first group of neurons described above can be divided into specific modes. That which is most discernible within an organism's consciousness is the perceptive mode (e.g., an accurate inner reconstruction of the sensory world). The second mode is reminiscent (e.g., recall of mental imagery), while the third is unconscious (e.g., deep sleep or anesthesia). The difference between these three modes is not technical in any way, but it is qualitative. The first relates to very accurate representations of the world and the conscious organism within it, and operates mainly in response to input from the senses. However, the same group of neurons could be involved in building up memory traces, that is, representing previously experienced events when the sensors are shut off or unattended. An extreme instance of this is sleep during which dreaming is taking place. Automata theory also shows that under certain conditions the machine enters states with a fairly random content. One of the pillars of *Impossible Minds* is that anything that is conscious must have some connection with world events or juxtapositions of world events. Random firing, or no firing at all, does not correlate with reported conscious experience, and this might constitute the automata theory definition of dreamless sleep or anesthesia.

Of course, learning is critical for an automaton to be able to "know" about the world it inhabits and senses. The iconic method described earlier in this chapter can easily be captured by automata theory. The inner states themselves are created by sensory input, but then become part of the state structure through the synaptic variations of the neurons. At first sight this is a bit hard to understand, but for the purposes of the current story it need not be fully understood. The enthusiast is referred to *Impossible Minds*. Suffice it to say here that iconic learning is a way of showing that the plasticity of neurons leads to inner firing patterns that represent the organism's world.

However, the patterns learned are not just static images of the world. Iconic learning can also result in the learning of sequences of events in the world. This allows the organism to recall the causes of events and their outcomes. It is through this process that the organism acquires its planning ability, because it acquires the ability to imagine alternative outcomes from its own actions. This predictive capability allows the organism to "know" the effect of its own actions on the world. In effect, this is like possessing models of the world which include one's own position and role in it: that is, a sense of self. The ability to predict outcomes, combined with a sense of self, leads to the ability to make choices; these could be constrained by personal need or could be free and arbitrary. This ability to make choices is equivalent to another vital element of consciousness: that is, will. An important corollary of all this is that it gives rise to differing personalities which are dependent on the choices made in the past.

It would be wrong to conclude that, in formulating *Impossible Minds*, I was only concerned with a kind of visual consciousness. Consciousness involves not only the five senses but a few internal and emotional ones as well. Therefore much of *Impossible Minds* is concerned with some of the interactions between these different sensory modalities. Thus I show that in considering the meaning of words one has to ask questions about how neural areas can create associations between different sensory representations—for instance, associating imagery with words. An important conclusion is that such representations have a logical structure which, for example, represents that "apple" is "fruit" but "fruit" is not "apple."

In this respect, automata theory and neural models enter one of the hottest debates of the last half of the twentieth century: the nature and origin of human language. This is a long story which, when cut short, makes a great deal of the learning of links between on the one hand iconic representations of the world and one's own actions in it, and on the other iconic representations of both written and spoken language. The conclusion is that we are not born with grammar in our heads, but that this is something that emerges through our need to transmit successes in our actions to others in the tribe. Nouns, verbs, other linguistic elements, and the linguistic structures that glue them together are a result of our ability to act on the world and to represent what we have done through complex, iconic neural firing. We shall meet a little more of this in chapter 12.

Impossible Minds would have been incomplete had it not considered how the analysis of neural automata impinges on what are regarded as the more abstract and mysterious elements of consciousness: qualia (the qualitative character of inner sensations); instincts; and emotions. Again, we shall meet qualia in chapter 12; but for the moment it is sufficient to say that, although the relationship between emotion and instinct appears to be amenable to neural automata analysis, the work still remains to be done.

Is MAGNUS Conscious?

In *Impossible Minds*, the answer given concerning MAGNUS's consciousness is, "Well, yes and no." "No" in the sense that a living organism is conscious of being a living entity, and therefore MAGNUS is not conscious like a human being; but "yes" in the sense that it might be conscious of being a machine and capable of telling us what it's like to be a machine. But more of this, too, in chapter 12.

More Possible Minds

The reader may get the impression that what has been discussed so far in this book is not very different from what was described in *Impossible Minds*. But a trip to California made me change my mind about one major thing: iconic learning. There is much less of it around than I thought. Here is part of the story.

California

In December 1996, I completed my period of rotation as head of the Electrical Engineering Department and was given a six-month sabbatical. On the suggestion of John Hopfield, Helen (who had a coincident sabbatical) and I went to the California Institute of Technology. This was an excellent experience. Luckily, just before I left, Barry Dunmall, who was then a visiting research fellow in my group, had completed an enormously flexible computing tool for building MAGNUS-like systems on ordinary PCs and laptops. These had advanced so much that more sophisticated models could be built on these machines than had been the case with the expensive laboratory version of MAGNUS. This meant that MAGNUS would easily come with me to California.

With Rodney Goodman I explored the possibility of actually building a robot version of MAGNUS. But this largely gave way to a project suggested by discussions with Christof Koch and a brief meeting with Francis Crick. I became convinced that one of the central features of consciousness was our visual awareness. The textbooks show over forty anatomical areas in the visual system associated with visual awareness. The brain operates on the basis of a subtle interplay between structures which have evolved so as to be effective, and learning which takes place within those structures. The ability of the visual system to create inner representations—that is, to see things—is an evolved property. What it makes of what it represents, and how it can imagine things it has never seen, require a more complex explanation than simple ideas about iconic learning provide.

At a seminar that I gave during a retreat of the Computation and Neural Systems group, I asked whether the anatomical and functional understanding of the visual system was sufficiently advanced to explain to me how I can visualize something I have never seen before—"a blue banana with red spots." The answer was negative, so this seemed an interesting quest. How does word-driven visualization work?

Ego-centered World Representations

So, explaining visual awareness came to the top of my research agenda. I continued working on this on my return to Europe and was able to show the beginnings of a model of the neurophysiology of a system capable of imagining things.

The main result obtained with MAGNUS was based on Chris Koch and Francis Crick's theories. Following closely the known anatomy of the visual system, I was able to show that a neural area could exist that coherently represents the world from the point of view of the observer. This receives signals both through visual channels and from the muscular activities of the system, giving it the capacity to reconstruct objects as they exist in the world but as seen from the point of view of the observer. We call this an "ego-centered world representation." This is in contrast to the images that fall on the retina of the eye and exist in the primary visual cortex. Those representations are "eye-centered" and are inconsistent with one another from moment to moment. The ego-centered area represents the world as it appears to be as an extension of oneself, rather than as it is captured by the eyes.

We have also been able to show that this area can reconstruct "mental images" from simple adjectival phrases (a blue circle or a yellow triangle). Indeed this system is capable of imagining "a blue banana with red spots" even if such an object has never been part of its learning experience. The way in which this happens is that the words stimulate specialist sensor-centered areas that represent blueness, red spottedness, and banananess, while the ego-centered world area does the rest. It is this ability to create these ego-centered representations that to my mind clinches what it is that a neural system needs as an essential engineering property in order to become visually aware.

These properties ending in "-ness" smack curiously of the "qualia" mentioned earlier: the qualitative feel of redness in a red circle, or the blueness of the sea on a sunny day. The first inklings that qualia emerged from the properties of sensor-centered areas in a system capable of visual awareness became the centerpiece of a lecture at the Royal Society on March 18, 1998. This means that it's time for me to attempt to bring together the many strands of the argument that have trailed through this book so far. I also need to elaborate on the importance of ego-centered world representation in almost all that is related to consciousness—whether in machines or living organisms.

12

On Being Conscious

The Ego in the Machine

A Denouement . . .

Were this a detective story, the last chapter ought to reveal "who dun it." Well, it is a *kind* of detective story because over the last eleven chapters I have been laying trails that suggest working with neural machines makes me feel that I understand my own consciousness. Now I need to be explicit as to why this is. The earlier chapters contain more than clues; they actually describe some of the key issues that have made an impression on me—be it philosophical or technological. Can this be wrapped into a neat equation, a formula, an ultimate statement? Regrettably, I would not be the first to come to the conclusion that there is no grand formula, no glittering prize, no startling revelation.

What there is, however, is a point of view from which a series of questions can be answered. The questions are all related to the personal puzzle raised in chapter 1. I now dub this the "Naive Question":

> What is there in my brain that allows me to feel that I, as an individual, live in a real world, can imagine without perception, know who I am, and am able to decide what I want to do?

In the rest of this chapter I wish to summarize how the experiences of which I have spoken in the earlier chapters give me faith in the progressive understanding from which some of the answers to the naive question are drawn.

Searle: Has He Blown the Philosophical Problem Out of the Water?

So far, I have talked of the American philosopher John Searle only in connection with his clear and welcome demolition of the idea that a programmed computer can develop an understanding of natural language (chapter 9). He has written many other important books in the last twenty years, and has always made an enormous amount of sense in pointing out the inconsistencies of many philosophical positions on the subject of consciousness. However, in his book *Mind, Language, and Society: Philosophy in the Real World*, I think that he draws a line under the philosophical discussion and opens the way to sound scientific investigation.

In summary, Searle draws attention to the need to have a fundamental belief in the fact that we live in a real world that exists in a way that is independent of our perception of it. While the likes of David Hume and George Berkeley (chapter 6) had the ingenious idea that there is no world reality but only that which is perceived, this is a position that blocks progress. It is a mistake of the kind that the philosophers of Miletus made in trying to develop a physics based on the premise that "all is water" or "all is air," which is only a first stab at discovering the real properties of matter (chapter 2).

In my work I assume that the world is real and that the more accurately a brain (real or artificial) brings this reality into the consciousness of the individual or the machine, the more successfully will that individual or machine cope with the real world.

The next quandary that Searle resolves is to lift constraints posed by classical "-isms" in philosophy. I am thinking of the dualism of Descartes (chapter 6) and the materialism of Daniel Dennett (of which a hint may be found in chapter 10). Searle sees these as default positions, which clash due to their mutual exclusivity. Helpfully, he suggests that the default positions should be ignored and that philosophies that take proper cognizance of both the dualist *and* materialist aspects of consciousness are likely to make general sense. That is, consciousness is a biologically generated phenomenon, and hence materialist; but it also gives the conscious organism personal sensations that appear to the organism to be independent of its biological machinery. In the same vein, he discounts the seeming impossibility of having a third-person (scientific) view of a first-person sensation, arguing again that it is for the biologist to discover which specific properties differentiate between being conscious and not.

The artificial consciousness of the artificial systems that I have been discussing in this book has precisely the characteristics of being capable of being seen as materialistic and dualistic. Being rooted in the material of a cellular architecture of many modules, artificial consciousness arises due to the representations of the world that emerge in such systems during both perception and imagination. Of which, more below . . .

Neural Systems and Ego-centered World Representation

Before attempting to attack the naive question, I shall recap what my experience of working with neural systems amounts to by returning to the idea of an ego-centered representation raised at the end of the last chapter. I assume that for a system to be conscious (or to be an artificial model within which consciousness can be studied), it must, as a necessary condition, possess neural machinery capable of creating ego-centered representations in some of its firing patterns. That is, through the firing of some neurons, it must have cellular areas within which states, or sequences of states, arise that represent the world the organism inhabits, as seen from the point of view of the organism. These states are generated through a highly specialized function of neural structures and their modification through learning. It seems to me evident that whenever neurons fire to contribute to states that reflect the cohesiveness of the world, one says that the organism "feels," "perceives," or "imagines" the world.

The phenomenon is vividly illustrated by what occurs when patterns of pin pricks in a finger activate neural states in the human somatosensory cortex that are coded for the exact position in which they exist on the surface of the body and "feel" to be not in the head but in the finger. This is an example of ego-centeredness that shows quite an astonishing effect. The "ego" in this neural activity, because it always locates events in the world (or the skin in this case), "feels" as if it is a vanishingly small center from which all observation takes place.

The reason this happens is that when something touches the tip of my finger, the firing of neurons due to this sensory input reaches the brain together with masses of other information deriving from the firing of neurons that transmit a vision of where the finger is. So were my finger to be touched a second time but with the fingertip displaced an inch or so from where it was the first time, part of the pattern of firing in my head would represent this difference. So the pinprick is represented in its appropriate position in space. But this implies a center from which these positions are measured. Hence our representations of the sensory world, by being fully representative of the origin in space of the stimulation, become ego-centered. That is, they put an unchanging entity I call "I" into my head. At the same time, there is no shortage of neurons in the cortex for these representations to have all the vivid detail of the real world.

The reader is encouraged to read V. S. Ramachandaran and Sandra Blakeslee's fascinating account of the way that patients whose arms have been amputated still have an "ego-centered" sensation of their fingers when the appropriate neurons in their cortex are stimulated.[2] This phenomenon provides an undeniable clue that neural firing patterns in the brain are reported by the owner of that brain as coming into consciousness in a way that encodes ego-centered representations of the world.

"Ego-centeredness" in the Visual System

To illustrate the very important idea of "ego-centered" inner states, I briefly return to some of the work that Barry Dunmall, Valentina Del Frate, and I have done on visual awareness, as was mentioned at the end of chapter 11.

Think of your two eyes and notice how, in order to update knowledge of where you are, they dart around. Your head may also move as you are gathering this information. Eyes are like peculiar cameras; the lens projects a somewhat distorted picture of the world onto the retina. This is where the firing of some neurons occurs, in the rods (which respond to light intensity) and the cones (which respond to color by each cell being specialized to fire on one of the basic colors). Were we to project these firing patterns on a screen, we should see a picture that is strangely distorted. We would not see any colors. Every time the eyes move, this picture would change completely, like a movie taken by a really bad cameraman. Were I looking at a red wall and then a green one, all that we would notice on the projection is that different groups of neurons fire—and this would be only in a small spot (the fovea) in the middle of the image. Indeed, only this tiny middle of the image would be anything like an accurate sample of the observed scene.

This is certainly *not* an ego-centered representation, but an eye-centered one. The task that the visual system performs so well is, first, to separate out the features of the retinal firing (color, intensity, edges, motion) in the early (occipital, or back of the skull) part of the visual system (the primary visual cortex, where things are still eye-centered). But our visual awareness, according to lesion experiments, appears to arise in deeper (frontal, or front of the skull) areas in the visual system, where neurons receive information from the firing of muscular neurons that control eye position and much else besides.[3] Here, maps may be created of shape information and color information which incorporate compensation for the position of the eye, the head, and even the motion of the body through space.

In a crude way we can think of the accurate part of the retina (the fovea) as being responsible for "painting" a neural picture on inner neural surfaces where the paintbrush is positioned by muscular signals that tell the brush where the fovea is. The *in*accurate part of the retina serves to attract the position of the paintbrush to things in the world that have content that is either important to the organism or is just changing. These "painted" surfaces are where ego-centered representations are created—and this is where visual awareness occurs.

The fact that several partial ego-centered representations coexist in areas that are separated from one another (shape, color, motion) hardly matters, because each of them is ego-centered. All areas in which this happens qualify for contributing to visual awareness. Areas do not qualify where the firing is eye-centered or system-centered without compensation being made for the activity of the organism.

I know that some neurophysiologists worry about how the different areas contributing to the ego-centered representation communicate with one another (they call it "the binding problem"). But I feel that this is not much of a problem because, to the owner of the neural structures, it does not matter much where the ego-centered neurons are; it is their ego-centered representation of the world that ensures the binding. That is, if a neuron in part A of my cortex is representing the edge of my green cup, and another in part

B is signaling that this edge is green, and both are world-representative and ego-centered, then they could coincide in my sensation of the event without actually communicating.

Interesting in this context is what happens if the connections in our brains start shifting around under abnormal conditions. I refer again to the work of Ramachandaran. He gives an absorbing account of what happens when the nerve endings of an amputee shift around to invade unused areas of the cortex: the patient feels that his fingers are being touched when, in fact, the side of his face is being stroked. The somatosensory neurons that would normally receive input from the tips of the fingers have now been "enervated" by face neurons that happen to be neighbors of the finger neurons in this part of the cortex. What better evidence could there be to tie down elements of consciousness to the firing of ego-centered neurons, which form the world of our tactile senses?

Ego-centered Representations: A Few Principles

I stress that it is the very ego-centeredness of some representations that distinguishes them as contributing to consciousness from other firing patterns that do not have this property. Firing in the neural system that keeps us breathing or keeps the heart active are examples of the latter. And so, indeed, is firing that may be driving ego-centered representations but is not ego-centered itself (such as firing in the retina and the primary visual cortex in vision).

It remains for the engineer working with the neurophysiologist to work out the details of how this enormously intricate system gets to create its ego-centered firing representations. This is available to hard-nosed analysis and modeling based on the broad mechanistic principles now known. It does not need a scientific revolution. In principle, we know how neural states can get to represent the world in sufficient detail and independently (unconsciously) of the effort needed to compensate for the peculiarities of the sensors (e.g., the movement of the eyes and the head in the case of vision). We also know in principle how these representations enable the organism to engage with precision and deliberation with that world using whatever output actuators (limbs, language, etc.) are at its disposal. And we know in principle how the system gets to have contemplative modes during which, without engaging with the world, its states follow state sequences that are ego-centered, either arbitrarily or according to some need, representing its ability to think.

With these principles in mind, I shall now try to answer some of the subsidiary puzzles that flow from our naive question.

Imagination?

In addition to showing in the artificial neural network that it is possible to get some insights into the way in which a brain might reconstruct reality, it has also been possible to show that it can imagine the world while not perceiving it. This evidently involves learning and language. Taking world representations of a visual kind, we note that they become linked to auditory (or visual) representations of names of things and actions. One can trigger the other when the other is not perceived. However, a most intriguing question we have been able to answer is "How does the brain construct things it has never seen?"

Before going further, the phrase "things it has never seen" needs to be qualified. I do not mean that the system is good at extrasensory perception and can guess what Abigail Witherspoon looks like without having ever seen her or heard her described. But a very good description might lead to the creation of a mental image that enables the imaginer to pick Abigail out in a crowd. Also, I could ask someone to imagine a flying pig or a pink elephant. What comes into consciousness is what is induced by the words.

Without going into technical detail, it appears possible that in learning to use words and language, neural links are established with areas that represent features such as colors or shapes, but that are not necessarily world-representative or ego-centered. It is the major emergent drive of the system to re-create the world that brings together partial and possibly unconscious representations of words, causing world-plausible representations to emerge. Of course, if there is no perception in any sensory domain, the inner networks can fall into "attractors" (which are meaningful states because they are created by perceptual experience) and allow us to imagine things seemingly at random. If this occurs during sleep, it is called dreaming.

Is It Just "Pictures in the Head"?

I am often asked whether this ego-centeredness is not just a variant of what Wittgenstein in his early writings called the "picture theory of the mind." Notably, this is a theory that he himself discredited in his later writings. In this theory, someone saying "cat" would cause some of my neurons to enter a state that is similar to the state they entered when a cat was seen and remembered.

Ego-centered representations do much more than just re-create pictures in my head. Simply they may re-create pictures, but they encode anything that is pertinent to the generators of those pictures in the world and the organism's relationship to such objects. The word *cup* creates neural representations not only of an image of the cup, but its ego-centeredness would include representations in motor areas of how I might grip the cup, how I might fill it, how I might drink from it, and how it might break if dropped. In other words, ego-centered representations encode my entire experience of what "cup" means to me! It encodes the "aboutness" of a cup. This is precisely the kind of process that John Searle had argued was missing in "hard" AI (chapter 9). Ego-centeredness in world representations, in Searle's language, means "incorporating intentionality."

To Be Conscious or to Have Consciousness?

Throughout this book I have maintained that much of the way that consciousness is being explained depends on the way that it has been discussed as a philosophical object. It was John Locke, the liberator of philosophy from dualism (chapter 6) who brought "consciousness" into philosophical discourse at the end of the seventeenth century. In 1904, William James (the "father" of psychology) reacted to the philosophy of the intervening three hundred years in a telling essay entitled "Does Consciousness Exist?"[4] His argument has much bearing on the way in which modeling using computers is being interpreted at the present time. His central thesis is that, while we can happily research the question of what it is to be or to become conscious, a belief that there is something called "consciousness" may be a misplaced use of words and could mislead the inquiry.

This mistake is present when it is suggested that a programmer could sit down and program "consciousness" into a computer. A program needs to be well understood by its creator, the programmer, and then inserted into a computer which "runs" or "has" that program. The detractors of conscious computers are quite right! A system could never become conscious through such a process. For ego-centered representations to emerge (i.e., for a system to become conscious), a system must interact with the world *and* have carefully designed physical structures. As William James rightly pointed out, speaking of "consciousness" could be the result of an inappropriate turning of an adjective into a noun, which is in turn interpreted as a possessible object. So this gives "consciousness" a possessible character that suggests that it is an object that can be donated to an otherwise unconscious entity. Wittgenstein (chapter 8) also warned us about such a mistake because it impinges on the word *having*. Even in the context of an event such as a toothache, one cannot *have* "a toothache" in the way one *has* "a new bicycle." In these terms, the programmer who writes the consciousness program and tries to make a computer possess it (or run it) may just have fallen into a linguistic trap!

How Does Emergence Resolve the Being/Having Problem?

Ways of "being" and "having" that would not offend William James apply when studying neural systems even through the use of computers. These can be illustrated with a room thermostat. A properly designed thermostat will gently correct the temperature of the room until it reaches the set point. A badly designed thermostat will cause the temperature to hunt about the set point. The first is stable and may appropriately be said to *have* stability. Now "stable" refers to a behavior of the system, while "stability" refers to its design and makeup. "Being stable" emerges for some set of conditions from the way that the system was designed—it was designed to "have stability" under many conditions.

So it is with artificial neural systems. The behavior of the system, or what the system is doing or representing at any point in time, emerges from the design of the network—that is, what the network *has*. But the design of the net has three major components: an initial structure guessed by the designer; improvements in this structure, which can be made when the performance of the system is observed (a kind of rapid evolution); and the ability of the structure itself to change through learning. In a very specific kind of neural system—the kind that people have in their heads—some of the design is made by a process of evolution and some by learning. So "being conscious" is that which emerges at a point in time and under some other conditions from the structural properties which the system "has"—that is, the structure that can represent ego-centered experience for many conditions and points in time. That could be called "having consciousness."

In neural systems engineering, it has always been the relationship between the structure of a neural system and its emergent properties that was at the center of what had to be discovered. In a study of consciousness, nothing has changed except ambition. It is the structure of neural systems that have the property of representing the world that needs to be understood. It is this effort that then throws light on the parallel problem in living nets of being conscious and having consciousness.

Why Do I Use Computers?

The programs that my colleagues and I write are not consciousness programs. They are programs that create neural laboratories within which the emergent properties of neural systems can be studied. The key target is to discover what, in simulated structures, gives rise to "ego-centered" representations of worlds that, in themselves, only exist as data inside a computer. In this way we hope to track down those architectural laws for the emergence of appropriate states that lead us to say things like "Aha, we now understand why the ratio of forward connections to reverse connections between area X of the visual system in the brain and area Y is what it is. Were it different, the ego-centered representation would not be sustained."

In other words, we use computers to get to grips with the complexities of neural structures in much the way that a weather forecaster uses computers to get to grips with the complexities of the weather. Nobody complains about the latter on the grounds of "computers cannot be the weather"; they only complain if it rains when fair weather is forecast.

Why Are Computer Scientists Skeptical of Emergent Properties?

Computer scientists generally react badly to a mention of emergent properties. "You have emergent properties," they quip, "when you don't know what your computer is doing!" This is a misunderstanding, or just a lack of willingness to consider the possibility of emergence in computation. A property is said to emerge from an interaction of active elements. This can happen in computation (and many people are interested in the properties of interacting "agents" in computer programs without recognizing that they have emergent properties). The quest in neural network studies is to understand how internal properties arise from structure and learning. Computer scientists have spent over fifty years in making sure that the structure of their machines does not influence what they want the machines to do. No wonder that any property arising from the structure of a machine is anathema (or, in computerese—a bug) to them. But the emergent properties in our studies are those of a program—a simulation—and not of a host computer.

So What Do Being Conscious and Having Consciousness Comprise?

At a superficial level, answering this question is suspiciously simple. Being conscious is perceiving accurately, remembering vividly, planning and acting, all on the basis of internal representations of the world and the placement of the organism within it, and—certainly not least—communicating with others. Having consciousness is having the technical capacity to code sensory signals into an accurate representation of the world and the role of the "self" within it, without which the seeing, perceiving, remembering, planning, and acting would not be possible.

What I am saying is that the real answer to the question at the head of this subsection lies in the detail of the function of neural systems, much of which still needs to be discovered. But, in broad principle, being conscious and having consciousness need not wait for a new form of science.

Is Every *Neural Network Therefore Conscious?*

Not in the least. In saying that being conscious is a property that emerges from a neural structure, all I am saying about neural nets is that, for me, this is an appropriate domain within which to investigate the phenomenon. There is a long way between this and saying something about what *kind* of emergent property being conscious might be and how well attuned the neural structures have to be to have consciousness. But to support the idea that working with neural networks is worthwhile, the next question needs to be asked.

Which Things Do We Think Are Conscious?

The problem with this question is that the answer depends on whom you ask. Purposefully excluding machines, we can go through a list, starting with human beings, who, most would argue, are the ultimate conscious inhabitants of the earth. However, the presence of consciousness among animals is a controversial issue.

On the whole, we are disposed to think of animals with bigger neural nets as being capable of being conscious. We would not give much chance for the consciousness of an amoeba, while we might be prepared to accept a chimp or a dolphin into the club, partly as a result of the similarity of their behavior to our own. But we would not class plants as having consciousness (despite the fact that some believe that they respond to kind conversation), for they have no nervous system. Of course, some believe that *only* humans are conscious. There is therefore a rough ordering between the sophistication of the neural system and the probability that an object may be conscious.

There is much controversy here too, and many would disagree with me about the above classification. Is a baby conscious? Or an embryo in its mother's womb? And what does "sophisticated" mean in the context of a neural system? The answers to such questions are not yet fully resolved, but I explore them in the next subsection.

Are There Different Kinds of Consciousness?

While I have no doubt that humans have reached some kind of pinnacle among the various forms of consciousness that might exist, I am equally sure that it is scientifically sound to allow that different kinds and levels of consciousness do actually exist. Part of the equation is what the organism needs to be, and is, conscious *of.* While an embryo may have progressively more apparatus available through which it will become conscious throughout its life, there may be very little scope for consciousness in its mother's womb. Consciousness, I have suggested, is an ego-centered representation of the world. In the womb the world is limited to the womb—which is, as a necessity of nature, welcoming, protective, and unchanging. So, while whatever consciousness there may be is ego-centered by definition, its content may be somewhat vacant. This means that the representation-building process may only begin in earnest after birth. I am not saying that the embryo is not conscious—the apparatus is progressively in place. I am merely saying that it is conscious of a very limited world with respect to what will happen later in life.

Applying this equation to a baby, there must be a bewildering amount of representation being built up as the world is laid out in all its splendor to be absorbed through the senses. Not only that, but much of the coordination that is needed to create ego-centered representations must begin to fall into place. This argument does not exclude structure that may be inborn (evolved) and which accelerates the process of absorbing representations.

Looking at the animal world, there seems to be little doubt that the perceptive part of being conscious is well catered for, but one is led to wonder about the powers of representation and visualization. While the jury may stay out on these issues for some time, it seems to me perverse to deny that part of whatever consciousness might be is present in all living species to a greater or lesser extent.

I would guess that animals have evolved with a good match between their survival needs and their ability to represent their worlds in a more or less sophisticated ego-centered way. For example, there is a belief now that a bee, with its 900,000 neurons, has an internal representation of a scene that holds promising pollen and that this stimulates its dance back at the hive where it communicates with other bees. When Colin Cherry talked about this in the 1950s, it was thought that the bee was just reacting in an automatic way to its return path from the pollen and its relationship to the sun.

What Difference Does Language Make?

One heck of a difference, I would say. Going into detail would lengthen this chapter by a few hundred pages. But the key issue is that in humans language is a powerful stimulant of inner representation. It is a well-trodden pathway that the success on Earth of human beings is due to the sophistication and accuracy with which the world can be internally represented, coupled with the ability to produce and be sensitive to a comprehensive repertoire of sounds.

The survival value of human tribes in prehistory must have been greatly enhanced by the coevolution of these two competencies, through the value of being able to transfer elements of ego-centered ideas about the world from one being to another. Being able to relate a bad experience with a poisonous mushroom and describing its subtle features to others in the tribe adds obvious survival value.

It is hardly surprising that, given the apparatus for both representation and generation, human beings in distant communities have developed languages that work in very similar ways. I would argue that they work so as to make as efficient as possible the rapid communication of ego-centered representations. The "language instinct," of which Steven Pinker speaks so eloquently, is much more bound up with, and controlled by, mechanisms that influence the creation of inner representations of the world than a specialized study of linguistics alone might reveal.[5]

The Self?

Where is the "self" in mechanistic or biological explanations of consciousness? It is a primary feature of the representational explanation that it essentially does *not* leave out the "I" in access to experience. That is precisely why it is so exciting to find *ego*-centered representations in systems which, as in our visual models, have the necessary modules and connections which also occur in the brain. Like the amputee's phantom arm, the representational activity in my brain intimately represents *my* arm, or *my* feelings. Even more intriguing is that a different twist in the neural system causes patients to disown parts of their body. It must be a distressing experience to live with an arm that feels as if it is someone else's but that follows you around all the time. (This is Ramachandaran's work again: see note 2, this chapter.)

Qualia?

Talk of "qualia" (the inner quality of sensation) leads to the conundrum of whether *my* experience of red is the same as *yours*. I need to put aside the fact that "the same" in this context may not be meaningful: what goes on in my head is by definition not "the same" as what goes on in yours, but it may be similar. Allowing that the question asks whether the same *mechanisms* are at work, the answer is clearly positive. Red is only meaningful in comparison with other experiences, and the shift in neural firing in the unconscious (early visual) representation between (say) redness and greenness comes into a world-centered representation together with other representations by what are likely to be the same mechanisms. A snapshot of my and your neurons thinking "red" would show nothing remarkable and might show considerable differences, but a shift to green in both our thoughts would show that neural activity has changed in both. Which is which is then nailed down by the association that these neural systems make with the representation of words in other parts of the brain.

Zombies?

Could there be zombies? That is, could one build an exact copy of a conscious being which was not conscious? According to ego-centered world-representing ideas, the answer is "no." If all the structures for ego-centered representations are in place and all the learned neural parameters are the same, the copy would not only be conscious but would think it was its generating prototype. However, were the neurons silicon rather than biological, there would at least be the difference that the zombie would soon become conscious of having silicon rather than biological needs. Outwardly, however, there may be little difference in behavior.

Third Person, First Person—Who Wins?

It is worth repeating the elegant question first asked by Thomas Nagel: "What is it like to be a bat?"[6] This points to the impossibility of knowing what it is like to be a bat, implying an impossibility of knowing what consciousness is like for any object outside oneself. Representational ideas suggest some necessary mechanisms for becoming conscious. Therefore, what I would look for in a bat are neural structures that would tell me about that bat's powers of representation. I could then make a series of statements such as, "Well, the scope in the bat for having language-driven representation is much more limited than mine. Its ego-centered representations are auditory." The better I understand how ego-centered representations come about, the more I will be able to take a guess about what it's like to be a bat in comparison with what it's like to be me.

These are factual statements. Totally knowing what it's like to be a bat is somewhat obviously predicted as being impossible by representational notions, because such experience is unavailable to my ego-centered representing neurons. However, extending this argument to saying that it is impossible to study consciousness in general through neural representation I think is a *non sequitur*.

How Conscious Could Machines Be?

Having accepted that the main reason for building neural machines with ego-centered representations is to study how such representations arise, once they *have* arisen, does this make the machine conscious? The classification I have given earlier of things that may or may not be conscious creates a single road between the amoeba and the human being. They are all living creatures.

So if we ask in what way a machine with the required mechanisms could be conscious, "Conscious of *what?*" may be a pertinent question. If I am in the Barbican Hall, London, listening to a symphony concert with Helen beside me, I would expect that she and I are conscious of much the same thing: the hall, the fullness of it, and many other visible and audible features. We may not be conscious of the music with a similar degree of pleasure: she may love it and I may hate it. She may be conscious of being thirsty and I of being hungry. Now, were a machine (looking much like an average Barbican Hall customer) be sitting on the other side of me, the chances are that, were it conscious at all, it could credibly be conscious of the physical features (which are shared by humans), but that might be all. Hunger and thirst, hate and love may not come into it. Need for electricity to charge up its batteries might.

The key difference between the machine and the person is that the machine would be conscious of being a machine, whereas the person is conscious of being a living human. It could lead to interesting conversations, provided that they both speak the same language. What I am saying is that a conscious machine (defined by its ego-centered representations) would be in a different plane from the amoeba-human line, but could still perceive, remember, plan, and communicate in its own machine-like way. Without its own appropriately tuned neural systems, however, it could not do these things.

What of Two and a Half Millennia of Philosophy?

The notion of ego-centered neural representation sounds simple enough. Do I have the temerity to suggest that it now should replace two and a half thousand years of philosophy, or even just the last three hundred years when the word *consciousness* has been used. Not at all: I am merely suggesting that the results coming from neurophysiology, coupled with neural modeling on computers, gives us some idea of what to look for in the brain when we wish to study the way that a brain generates consciousness.

Personally, I find it hard to forget the philosophy that has always acted as a guide to the very complexity of the subject. It is this complexity that has prompted some of the greatest minds in history to face the subject without the benefit of scientific support. Imagine trying to discuss radio broadcasts without the concept of electromagnetic propagation, or the flight of a jumbo jet with no knowledge of aerodynamic theory or the workings of a jet engine. No wonder that mystique and disagreement pervade the philosophical history of the subject.

But all this still means that the methods of the Miletians, the purity of Greek logic, the practicality of the empiricists, the puzzled thoughts of Wittgenstein, and the disagreements of the present day are very much a part of the fascination of consciousness. It is hoped that what comes from the artificial domain adds a factual element to the debate.

The Future?

I think that things are changing, in the sense that analysis and modeling are beginning to get a grip on how our brains make us conscious. All that this means is that the subject of consciousness may, in a few years' time, no longer be of interest to philosophers. But for the neuroscientist and the neuroengineer the story is only just beginning.

To those who believe that science is not sufficiently developed to give us an answer now, but will some day yield the glittering truth, I say that they may be waiting unnecessarily. Like the alchemists of the past, they may be hunting for the golden formula, where the hard-nosed chemistry that gives a less dazzling answer is in clear evidence.

To those who believe that science can never explain the personal nature of our sensations even when the neural functioning of the brain has been fully understood, I say that they may be retelling cultural stories, which is dictated by a need for self-esteem—as was the ancient need to believe that the Earth was at the center of the universe. The emotional appeal of there being a "hard problem" out there that will forever be outside the grasp of science is akin to the notion that it is the poet's use of the word *heart* that tells us what "heart" is. I thoroughly enjoy good poetry, but were I dragged into a hospital after a heart attack I would rather see a cardiac surgeon than a poet.

To those who feel that I am blaspheming by treating as material that which religions have held to be divinely created, I say that they may be making a mistake. As Galileo's *eppur si muove* (and yet it moves) was seen as blasphemy, the error was that of men and not of any divinity. Any robust theology should not be offended by logical argument. If I feel that a material explanation of my own consciousness is more satisfactory than what theology can deliver, this is good news for theology: one less thing to worry about. Most devout people in the Judeo-Christian tradition do not believe in literal interpretations of the Testaments of their religions, accepting more earthy arguments. This does not diminish the role of theology—there is still much unknown, for which religious belief provides comfort for some: I am thinking of the death of a loved friend, the unfairness of human ambition, and the cruelty of natural disasters.

What I have set out here are bold statements, and perhaps I have not earned my stripes for making them. But for me the naive personal question is beginning to get some answers—answers that, I hope, also make sense to others.

Epilogue—2100

Conscious Systems
The Last Lecture

The scene: Galactic College, London, June 2100.
The lecturer: Professor Ravishnar Ponsenby, 60, the noted designer of MOLECULA 16, the world's first conscious machine, built in 2070.

PROFESSOR: Thank you all for coming to this face-to-face lecture, and thank you for attending the lectures in the past from your own universe net stations. What I want to do is just mull over some of the most important points that have been made during the course itself.

STUDENT 1: Is that because they will be on the examination?

PROFESSOR: Now Johnstone, exams . . . exams. That's all that seems to matter to you. Don't you care about the things we have been discussing? The ideas . . . the theories . . . the philosophy? Anyway, surely you don't expect me to answer your question.

STUDENT 1 TO STUDENT 2 *(SOTTO VOCE)*: It will be on the exam . . .

PROFESSOR: The first point is historical. You have to know why so many philosophers—until the first decade of this millennium— were so insistent that science could not approach the problem of consciousness.

STUDENT 3: Why was it, Professor Ponsenby?

PROFESSOR: Are you trying to get me angry, Tong Yie? I am suggesting that when you get home this evening you take your watch-computer out, plug into the wall-screen, and take a good look at your course materials. Then get some of this stuff into that skull of yours. You will discover that philosophers at the end of the last millennium were determined just to talk things out. But they had to give this up, because as the answer lies in the emergent properties of neural systems, the younger generation in philosophy demanded that they be taught sufficient mathematics to understand the automata theory that interdisciplinary teams in the neurosciences were using. This returned philosophy to its pre-Lockean position of requiring a good grasp of mathematics and the sciences.

Then you will recall that the new super brain-scans revealed that, indeed, the world was represented as ego-centered neural firing patterns. This confirmed the theoretical conclusions that had been postulated right at the beginning of the millennium.

STUDENT 4: Why was MOLECULA 16 a failure?

PROFESSOR: Why do you think it was a failure? It never went to Mars, which was the task it was designed for, but that was due to cuts in the space program. But it still does a good job flying the commercial shuttle service to the Moon—indeed, it is probably the safest way of flying that shuttle. The fact that it will be replaced by a human astronaut is so as to have equality across the flying force. The transport company wants to demonstrate that humans are just as good as conscious robots simply because they cannot afford to build more MOLECULA robots.

STUDENT 4: But I hear that it is going into the Delhi national museum. Won't it get bored?

PROFESSOR: Now Carmen, this is something that we talked about during the lectures, emotions in conscious machines.

STUDENT 4: Did we?

PROFESSOR: I did explain that emotional representations in MOLECULA were only of the basic visceral kind: fear and pleasure. Being in the museum and talking to visitors will simply give MOLECULA a sense of mild pleasure for fulfilling her current mission.

STUDENT 4: But will it not feel that it is a failure? Would it not have looked forward to going to Mars? Would it not be disappointed?

PROFESSOR: You are doing just what I spent much time telling you not to do: confusing human emotions with machine emotions. MOLECULA has no personal agenda because she is not competing with anyone. Emotions such as "disappointment" at not doing something that a human would be proud of and that would make that human feel more attractive in his society are just totally inappropriate for a machine. But threaten its memory and you will get a long lecture about wasting investment and training time.

STUDENT 5: Could it fall in love with some of the visitors?

PROFESSOR: I shall not answer this—work it out for yourself. Think about what I have said regarding inappropriate emotions.

STUDENT 4: How do you know that MOLECULA will not get fed up and start getting nasty to people just for amusement?

PROFESSOR: I see that much of my course was wasted on you. Consciousness does not mean that the conscious machine will acquire all the weaknesses of a human being. Consciousness does not mean humanity—that's Law 1. If you know nothing else you should know this. But, conversely, humanity has been successful entirely through being conscious.

STUDENT 3: Are there any good research jobs in your team?

PROFESSOR: That depends, Tong Yie. It depends on the grades you get on this course among other things. But, given that all of that goes well, I do have a grant to implement some of our ideas on artificially conscious machines for language understanding. Despite all our demonstrations that systems could understand stories in the full sense of the word, the computer networking providers are still looking for the design of net agents that could have a really intimate understanding of the needs of specific net users. There are several things of that kind that we have been asked to research: artificial videophone operators that understand the queries of visitors, and fully comprehending primary-care medical systems.

STUDENT 3: Oh, Professor, do you not have anything that has to do with games? I hear that artificial consciousness is being applied to dolls that get depressed if you don't speak to them lovingly.

PROFESSOR: Now I totally disapprove of such ideas. They use the human power of attributing feelings to nonliving objects in a totally inappropriate way. They have to hide the real mechanical nature of the doll. It is deception on a grand scale.

STUDENT 6: How much do we need to know about the latest automata-theory analyses of ego-centered representations? Particularly, I don't understand the mathematics in your papers. I don't think that I understand any of it!

PROFESSOR: This, Vipna Fernandez, brings me neatly to the last point of this brief meeting. I am disappointed that you understand so little, but maybe you are approaching it in the wrong way. Forget the jargon, forget the equations and the mathematics that you read in our papers. Our peers who review our papers have this strange idea that mathematical ways of describing things gives them a special legitimacy. All you have to realize is that the artificial brains that have been developed since the turn of the millennium, things like MAGNUS, and the mathematical analyses are only tools that are meant to give us as good an understanding as possible of our own conscious brains. So the issue of understanding what goes on does not depend on your ability to do mathematics, so long as you accept that the artificial consciousness in MAGNUS tells us something about the real thing. It is this same understanding that leads to the creation of artificially conscious robots such as MOLECULA.

STUDENT 6: So what's the first thing I need to understand?

PROFESSOR: All that automata theory tells you is that the behavior of the system is mainly dependent on the internal state that the internal connections between the neurons get into. Learning means creating states that are stable and related to experience. But the brain has lots and lots of these machines with internal states; and most of the books and papers on the subject tell you what, in the brain, these boxes are representing. The main conclusion is that some of these boxes are so full of neurons that they represent the world as it is, including the point of view of the observer. The reason that talking of these things falling in love is nonsense is because an artificial system can have the representations, but they are colored by their own machine-like character. Have I used any mathematics? All you have to do is to elaborate on the many points I have now glossed over.

STUDENT 1 TO STUDENT 2 (*SAME SOTTO VOCE*): Good old Vipna. Now we know what's on the exam . . .

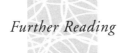

Further Reading

Neural System Technology
Aleksander, Igor and Helen Morton. *Introduction to Neural Computing.* London: Thompson International Press, 1995.

Neural Modeling of Thought
Aleksander, Igor. *Impossible Minds: My Neurons, My Consciousness.* London: Imperial College Press, 1996.

Biographies in Neural Networks
Anderson, James and Edward Rosenfeld. *Talking Nets: An Oral History of Neural Networks.* Cambridge: MIT Press, 1998.

A Critical History of Philosophy
Russell, Bertrand. *A History of Western Philosophy* (1961). Rpt., New York: Simon and Schuster, 1975.

General Texts on the Mind
Blakemore, Colin. *The Mind Machine.* London: BBC Books, 1998.
Gregory, Richard, ed. *The Oxford Companion to the Mind.* New York and Oxford: Oxford University Press, 1987.

Consciousness
Chalmers, David J. *The Conscious Mind: In Search of a Fundamental Theory.* Oxford: Oxford University Press, 1996.

Crick, Francis. *The Astonishing Hypothesis: The Scientific Search for the Soul.* New York: Scribner's, 1994.

Dennett, Daniel. *Consciousness Explained.* Boston: Little Brown, 1991.

Penrose, Roger. *Shadows of the Mind: A Search for the Missing Science of Consciousness.* New York and Oxford: Oxford University Press, 1994.

Cognition

Bruce, Vicki, ed. *Unsolved Mysteries of the Mind: Tutorial Essays in Cognition.* New York: Psychology Press, 1995.

Memory

Rose, Steven. *The Making of Memory* (1992). Rpt., Garden City, N.Y.: Doubleday Anchor, 1993.

Neurology

Ramachandaran, V. S. and Sandra Blakeslee. *Phantoms in the Brain: Human Nature and the Architecture of Mind.* New York: William Morrow, 1998; pbk., New York: Quill, 1999.

Notes

Preface

1. Eric Laithwaite was a professor at Imperial College, London University, who pioneered the linear motor, which led to electromagnetically levitated monorail trains. Many will remember him for his televised Christmas lectures at the Royal Institution. His passionate interest in the engineering feats of nature can be enjoyed in his book *An Inventor in the Garden of Eden* (Cambridge: Cambridge University Press, 1994).

I. Imagination and Consciousness

1. In 1980, John Searle wrote a celebrated paper suggesting that computers process but do not understand natural language: "Minds, Brains, and Programs," *Behavioural and Brain Sciences* 3 (1980): 417–24.

2. D. J. Chalmers, *The Conscious Mind: In Search of a Fundamental Theory* (Oxford: Oxford University Press, 1996).

3. One of the main advocates of the current inadequacy of science is Roger Penrose. His two books on consciousness are very clear on this point: *The Emperor's New Mind* (1989; rpt., New York: Penguin, 1991) and *Shadows of the Mind: A Search for the Missing Science of Consciousness* (New York: Oxford University Press, 1994).

4. John Searle, *Mind, Language, and Society: Philosophy in the Real World* (1999; pbk. rpt., New York: Basic Books, 2000).

3. Nineteen Fifty-eight: A Voyage Toward Interdisciplinarity

1. An excellent introduction to the history of the study of the mind is H. Gardner's *The Mind's New Science* (New York: Basic Books, 1985).

2. Norbert Wiener, *Cybernetics* (Cambridge: MIT Press, 1947).

3. Norbert Wiener, *The Human Use of Human Beings*. Originally published by MIT Press in 1950, this is now available in the Da Capo Series in Science (1988).

4. Chapter 8 in *Cybernetics* is a far-sighted essay not only on the theory of communication but also on the effect that the control of information has on the fortunes of society.

4. The Ghost of Aristotle: An Influence Across Two Millennia

1. Exceptionally, in 1999, during the writing of this book, I gave public lectures in India. Here, there were refreshing questions that were clearly not part of the Aristotelian tradition. These differed, but the notion of meditation, which strives to lead the mind of an individual to become part of a divine unknown, was confirmation that the high value a person places on their ability to think is truly universal.

2. The philosophical background to this chapter comes from two sources. The first is Bertrand Russell's *History of Western Philosophy* (1961; rpt., New York: Simon and Schuster, 1975), quoted in chapter 2. Another useful book is *The Mind*, by Daniel Robinson (Oxford: Oxford University Press [Oxford Readers], 1998. This contains original writings of Aristotle, Saint Thomas Aquinas, and Saint Augustine.

3. The historical background to Aristotle and Alexander may be found in *The Rise of the Greeks* by Michael Grant (New York: Collier Books, 1989).

5. Early Artificial Neurons and the Beginnings of Artificial Intelligence

1. John von Neumann, *The Computer and the Brain* (published posthumously in 1958 from von Neumann's 1955 Stillman Lectures at Yale University; rpt., 2d ed., New Haven: Yale University Press, 2000).

2. Michael Arbib, *Brains, Machines, and Mathematics*, 2d ed. (New York: Springer-Verlage, 1987).

3. Many books have been written on the history of computers. A textbook that provides a clear overview is *Computer: A History of the Information Machine* by Martin Campbell Kelly and William Aspray (New York: HarperCollins, 1997).

4. The classic paper by Claude Shannon is "Programming a Computer to Play Chess," *Philosophy* 41 (1950): 356–75. A more accessible description of Shannon's program may be found in "Automatic Chess Player," *Scientific American* (October 1950): 48.

5. A highly descriptive account of the rise of Artificial Intelligence, seen from the point of view of U.S. developments, is *The Age of Intelligent Machines*, ed. Ray Kurzweil (Cambridge: MIT Press, 1990). A more technical account but also written for the nonspecialist is by Margaret Boden: *Artificial Intelligence and Natural Man* (New York: Basic Books, 1977).

6. W. S. McCulloch and W. Q. Pitts, "A Logical Calculus of the Ideas Immanent in Neural Networks," *Bulletin of Mathematical Biophysics* 5 (1943): 115–33.

6. Liberating Philosophy: The Empiricists

1. Descartes's *Meditations on First Philosophy* are reproduced in the Cambridge Texts in the History of Philosophy, edited by John Cottingham (Cambridge: Cambridge University Press, 1996).

2. A concise presentation of Locke's philosophy is in Michael Ayres's *Locke: Ideas and Things* (New York: Routledge, 1999).

3. Another concise treatment, this time of Hume's philosophy, can be found in *Hume* by Anthony Quinton (1998; rpt., New York: Routledge, 1999).

4. *The Cambridge Companion to Kant*, ed. Paul Guyer (Cambridge: Cambridge University Press, 1992), is a multiauthored view of this most important philosopher.

7. Canterbury: The First Machines

1. Alan Turing, "Computing Machines and Intelligence," *Mind* 59 (1950): 433–60.

2. Frank Rosenblatt of Cornell University wrote *Perceptrons: An Introduction to Neurodynamics* (New York: Spartan, 1962) during a period of

instability in the development of computer theory. Logic was the favored approach and Rosenblatt's use of statistics was treated with suspicion.

3. Marvin Minsky and Seymour Papert put mathematical flesh on the unpopularity of Rosenblatt's approach by writing *Perceptrons: An Introduction to Computational Geometry* (Cambridge: MIT Press, 1969).

4. Computers also have magnetic storage—that is, hard disk or floppy diskettes for storing software and the products of applications. This is very capacious: 8,000,000,000 bytes (8 gigabytes) is standard hard-disk capacity for a desktop computer in 1999. This takes several noticeable seconds to access. RAM is fast and used for the actual computations of the machine, and it only takes small fractions of a millionth of a second to access.

5. The *Parallel Distributed Processing* books, edited by David Rumelhart and Jay McClelland, became bestsellers (Cambridge: MIT Press, 1986).

6. J. J. Hopfield, "Neural Networks and Physical Systems with Emergent Collective Computational Abilities," *Proceedings of the National Academy of Sciences (USA)* 79 (1982): 2554–58; and Hopfield, "Neurons with Graded Response Have Collective Computational Properties Like Those of Two-state Neurons," *Proceedings of the National Academy of Sciences (USA)* 81 (1984): 3088–92.

7. See notes at the end of chapter 5 (above) for references to the development of AI.

8. Stuart Kauffman has reflected recently on this problem in his book *The Origins of Order, Self-Organization, and Selection in Evolution* (New York: Oxford University Press, 1993).

8. Wittgenstein: A Brief Interlude

1. Bertrand Russell, *The Autobiography of Bertrand Russell* (1998 reissue ed.; pbk., New York: Routledge, 2000).

2. Ray Monk, *Wittgenstein: The Duty of Genius* (New York: Penguin, 1991).

3. David J. Chalmers, *The Conscious Mind: In Search of a Fundamental Theory* (Oxford: Oxford University Press, 1996).

9. The WISARD Years: Machines with No Mind

1. Peter Large, *The Micro Revolution* (pbk., New York: St. Martin's, 1981).

2. Michael Eysenck and Mark Keane, *Cognitive Psychology: A Student's Handbook*, 4th ed. (New York: Psychology Press, 2000).

3. Glyn Humphreys and Vicki Bruce, *Visual Cognition* (New York: Psychology Press, 1989).

4. James Lighthill, *A Report on Artificial Intelligence* (London: UK Science and Engineering Research Council, 1973).

5. A useful "insider" description of the Alvey program has been written by the director of the program, Brian Oakley. It appears as "Intelligent Knowledge-based Systems: AI in the UK," in Ray Kurzweil, ed., *The Age of Intelligent Machines* (Cambridge: MIT Press, 1990).

6. Searle, "Minds, Brains, and Programs," *Behavioural and Brain Sciences* 3 (1980): 417–24.

10. Starting the Week with Consciousness

1. Melvyn Bragg is a TV and radio personality in Britain as well as a historian with a strong interest in science and scientists. His book *On Giants' Shoulders* (1998; rpt., New York: John Wiley, 1999), based on a series of radio programs, discusses the past and future of science.

2. A recent book by Susan Greenfield is *The Human Brain* (1997; pbk., New York: Basic Books, 1998).

3. Roger Penrose explains his views on consciousness in *Shadows of the Mind: A Search for the Missing Science of Consciousness* (New York: Oxford University Press, 1994).

4. Steven Rose has written (among many other books) the prize-winning *The Making of Memory* (1992; rpt., New York: Doubleday Anchor, 1993).

11. MAGNUS in South Kensington and Pasadena

1. Jasia Reichardt, in *Frankenstein, Creation and Monstrosity*, ed. Stephen Bann (London: Reaktion Books, 1995).

2. J. J. Hopfield, "Neural Networks and Physical Systems with Emer-

gent Collective Computational Abilities," *Proceedings of the National Academy of Sciences (USA)* 79 (1982): 2554–58; and Hopfield, "Neurons with Graded Response Have Collective Computational Properties Like Those of Two-state Neurons," *Proceedings of the National Academy of Sciences (USA)* 81 (1984): 3088–92.

3. See note 5, chapter 7 (above).

4. Roger Penrose, *The Emperor's New Mind* (1989; rpt., New York: Penguin, 1991).

5. Daniel Dennett, *Consciousness Explained* (Boston: Little Brown, 1991).

6. Francis Crick, *The Astonishing Hypothesis: The Scientific Search for the Soul* (New York: Scribner's, 1994).

7. Igor Aleksander, *Impossible Minds: My Neurons, My Consciousness* (London: Imperial College Press, 1996).

12. On Being Conscious: The Ego in the Machine

1. Searle, *Mind, Language, and Society: Philosophy in the Real World* (1999; pbk. rpt., New York: Basic Books, 2000).

2. V. S. Ramachandaran and Sandra Blakeslee, *Phantoms in the Brain: Human Nature and the Architecture of Mind* (New York: William Morrow, 1998; pbk., New York: Quill, 1999.

3. Francis Crick and Christof Koch, "The Problem of Consciousness," *Scientific American* (September 1992): 153–56.

4. William James, "Does Consciousness Exist?" Reprinted in *The Writings of William James*, ed. J. J. McDermott (Chicago: University of Chicago Press, 1977).

5. Steven Pinker, *The Language Instinct* (1994; pbk., Harper Perennial Library 1995).

6. Thomas Nagel, "What Is It Like to Be a Bat?" *Philosophical Review* 4 (1974): 435–50.

Index

abstractions, 79
"Adaline," 144
Adaway, Bill, 125
AI. *See* artificial intelligence
   (AI)
air, 24–25
Aleksander, Igor: academic career,
   4, 6, 29–30, 33, 57–59, 70,
   87–88, 102–103, 114–15,
   126, 145–46, 157; as British
   Cybernetics Society President,
   35; Colin Cherry Memorial
   Lecture, 151–52; conversation
   with Dunmall, vii–viii; *The
   Human Machine*, 103; on
   imagined *Start the Week*, 134;
   Impossible Minds, 152–56; industrial experience, 33; leaving
   South Africa, 29–30; personal
   life, 101, 121; present from
   Uncle Dragutin, 30; on religion, 44; seasickness of, 30;
   talk at Trinity College, Cam-

bridge, 105; visit to MIT,
   99–101
Alexander of Macedon, 45, 46,
   50–52
Alvey, John (Alvey program),
   118
Amari, Shun Ichi, 145
amputees, 165, 167, 176
Anaximander, 7, 19, 20–24, 26
Anaximenes, 7, 17–20, 24–25,
   26
Ancient Greece, 7–8, 15–28,
   44–54
Anderson, James, 144
AND gates, 36, 70
a priori knowledge, 81, 82
Arbib, Michael, 57
Aristotle, 8, 44–54
artificial intelligence (AI), 4–5, 65,
   99, 120–21; Lighthill report
   on, 116–18
Ash, Sir Eric, 145, 146
assembly language, 62